The KEY TOPICS Series

Advisors:

T.M. Craft *Department of Anaesthesia and Intensive Care, Royal United Hospital, Bath, UK*
C.S. Garrard *Intensive Therapy Unit, John Radcliffe Hospital, Oxford, UK*
P.M. Upton *Department of Anaesthetics, Royal Cornwall Hospital, Treliske, Truro, UK*

Anaesthesia, Second Edition

Obstetrics and Gynaecology, Second Edition

Accident and Emergency Medicine

Paediatrics, Second Edition

Orthopaedic Surgery

Otolaryngology

Ophthalmology

Psychiatry

General Surgery

Renal Medicine

Trauma

Chronic Pain

Oral and Maxillofacial Surgery

Oncology

Cardiovascular Medicine

Neurology

Neonatology

Gastroenterology

Thoracic Surgery

Forthcoming titles include:

Respiratory Medicine

Orthopaedic Trauma Surgery

Critical Care

Accident and Emergency Medicine, Second Edition

A CIP catalogue record for this book is available from the British Library.

ISBN 1 85996 155 X

BIOS Scientific Publishers Ltd
9 Newtec Place, Magdalen Road, Oxford OX4 1RE, UK
Tel. +44 (0)1865 726286. Fax. +44 (0)1865 246823
World Wide Web home page: http://www.bios.co.uk/

Important Note from the Publisher
The information contained within this book was obtained by BIOS Scientific Publishers
Ltd from sources believed by us to be reliable. However, while every effort has been
made to ensure its accuracy, no responsibility for loss or injury whatsoever occasioned
to any person acting or refraining from action as a result of information contained herein
can be accepted by the authors or publishers.

The reader should remember that medicine is a constantly evolving science and while
the authors and publishers have ensured that all dosages, applications and practices are
based on current indications, there may be specific practices which differ between
communities. You should always follow the guidelines laid down by the manufacturers
of specific products and the relevant authorities in the country in which you are
practising.

Production Editor: Jonathan Gunning.
Typeset by J&L Composition Ltd, Filey, UK.
Printed by T.J. International Ltd, Padstow, UK.

CONTENTS

CONTRIBUTORS

Chris Compeau MD MSc FRCSC
Assistant Professor of Surgery, University of Toronto, Ontario, Canada

Gail Darling MD FRCSC
Assistant Professor of Surgery, University of Toronto, Ontario, Canada

Ziv Gamliel MD MSc FRCSC
Assistant Professor of Surgery, University of Maryland, Baltimore, MD, USA

Fang Gao MB BS MPhil FRCA
Consultant Anesthetist, Birmingham Heartlands Hospital, Birmingham, UK

Sean Grondin MD FRCSC
Chief Resident, Thoracic Surgery, University of Toronto, Ontario, Canada

Renee Kennedy MD FRCSC
Chief Resident, Thoracic Surgery, University of Toronto, Ontario, Canada

Shaf Keshafjee MD MSc FRCSC
Assistant Professor of Surgery, University of Toronto, Ontario, Canada

Donna E. Maziak MD FRCSC
Assistant Professor of Surgery, University of Ottawa, Ontario, Canada

Hani K. Najm FRCS
Fellow, Cardiovascular Surgery, University of Toronto, Ontario, Canada

F. Griff Pearson MD FRCSC
Professor of Surgery, University of Toronto, Ontario, Canada

Simon Pickard FRCS
Senior House Officer, Thoracic Surgery, Birmingham Heartlands Hospital, Birmingham, UK

ABBREVIATIONS

ABC	airway, breathing, circulation
ACTH	adrenocorticotrophic hormone
ADH	anti-diuretic hormone
AIDS	acquired immune deficiency syndrome
AP	antero-posterior
APUD	amine precursor uptake and decarboxylase
ARDS	adult respiratory distress syndrome
BAC	bronchioloalveolar carcinoma
CBC	complete blood count
CCAM	congenital cystic adenomatoid malformation
CMV	controlled mandatory ventilation
CNS	central nervous system
CO_2	carbon dioxide
COPD	chronic obstructive pulmonary disease
CPAP	continuous positive airway pressure
CT	computed tomography
CVP	central venous pressure
CXR	chest X-ray
D_LCO	carbon monoxide diffusing capacity
DLT	double-lumen endotracheal tube
ECMO	extracorporeal membrane oxygenation
EGJ	esophagogastric junction
EKG	electrocardiogram
ENT	ear, nose and throat
F	French scale
FEV_1	forced expiratory volume in one second
FiO_2	fractional inspired oxygen tension
FVC	forced vital capacity
GERD	gastroesophageal reflux disease
GI	gastrointestinal
GU	genitourinary
Gy	gray (one joule of energy/kg tissue)
HCG	human chorionic gonadotrophin
HC1	hydrochloric acid
HFJV	high frequency jet ventilation
HFO	high frequency oscillation
HFPPV	high frequency positive pressure ventilation
HLA	human leukocyte-associated antigen
IMV	intermittent mandatory ventilation
IU	international units
IV	intravenous
IVC	inferior vena cava
kPa	kiloPascals
LDH	lactate dehydrogenase

LES	lower esophageal sphincter
LVRS	lung volume reduction surgery
MFH	malignant fibrous histiocytoma
mM	millimol
mmHg	millimetres mercury
MRI	magnetic resonance imaging
MUSE	metaplasia ulcers stricture erosions
Nd-YAG	neodymium–yttrium aluminum garnet
NPO	nil by mouth
NSAID	non-steroidal anti-inflammatory drug
NSCLC	non-small cell lung cancer
NSE	neuron-specific enolase
O_2	oxygen
OLV	one-lung ventilation
PA	postero-anterior
$PaCO_2$	carbon dioxide tension in arterial blood
PaO_2	oxygen tension in arterial blood
PAS	periodic acid–Schiff
PCA	patient controlled analgesia
PCI	prophylactic cranial irradiation
PCR	polymerase chain reaction
PCWP	pulmonary capillary wedge pressure
PEEP	positive end expiratory pressure
PET	positron emission tomography
PSV	pressure support ventilation
PTFE	polytetrafluoroethylene
RA	right atrium
RR	respiratory rate
RV	right ventricle
SaO_2	oxygen saturation
SCLC	small cell lung cancer
SIMV	synchronized intermittent mandatory ventilation
SVC	superior vena cava
SVCO	superior vena caval obstruction
Tc	technetium
TNM	tumor node metastasis
UES	upper esophageal sphincter
VATS	video-assisted thoracoscopic surgery
VIP	vasoactive intestinal polypeptide
VMA	vanillyl mandelic acid
VO_2max	maximal oxygen uptake
V/Q	ventilation/perfusion
V_T	tidal volume

PREFACE

After over three decades of domination by cardiac surgery, general thoracic surgery has re-emerged as a distinct specialty. In some countries, separate specialty certification is now offered. Because of this growing recognition of the discipline, training in thoracic surgery has been re-focused. Now, more than ever, trainees in thoracic surgery, general surgery, cardiac or cardiothoracic surgery are being tutored by dedicated thoracic surgeons. Professional organizations, journals and textbooks are now beginning to reflect this new focus.

This book is primarily aimed at those postgraduate trainees who require thoracic surgery as a component of their certification examinations. This includes trainees in general thoracic surgery, cardiac or cardiothoracic surgery, and general surgery. It should be used in conjunction with larger, more comprehensive texts, when further detail is needed for any of the key topics highlighted. This book should also be a useful quick reference for senior medical students, clinical clerks, and those paramedical personnel such as nurses, physiotherapists and respiratory therapists, who play such a crucial role in the management of thoracic surgical patients.

In the text, we have tried to include all of the current key topics relevant to modern general thoracic surgical practice. Each chapter is limited to several pages of concise information presented in short note-form. Most of the topics were written by senior thoracic residents in conjunction with junior and senior faculty of the Division of Thoracic Surgery at the University of Toronto. The text was then formatted extensively by the editors to provide consistency and quick reference for the busy young clinicians who hopefully will benefit from it.

We are extremely grateful for the assistance of Frances Hui (Mount Sinai Hospital, Toronto), Kelly Dolson and Dianne Russell (Birmingham Heartlands Hospital), for the critical comments of Dr Valerie Rusch (Memorial Sloan Kettering Cancer Center, New York) on the manuscript, for the help of Dr Ruth Cayton (Birmingham Heartlands Hospital) in reviewing selected topics ('Bullous disease and emphysema' and 'Pulmonary function studies'), and for the expert help, encouragement and most of all patience, of Dr. Jonathan Ray, Managing Director of BIOS Scientific Publishers.

A. G. Casson
M. R. Johnston

ACHALASIA

Donna E. Maziak, F. Griff Pearson

Achalasia is an uncommon motility disorder of the esophagus, with an estimated incidence of 1 case per 100 000 population. It is most commonly diagnosed in the third decade of life.

Pathophysiology

Primary achalasia is thought to represent a degenerative nerve process, with characteristic histopathologic changes comprising loss of ganglion cells in the myenteric plexus and a reduction in vagal nerve fibers within the wall of the esophagus. The resulting physiologic alterations [i.e. failure of relaxation of the lower esophageal sphincter (LES) and ineffective peristalsis in the body of the esophagus] are thought to lead to hypertrophy of the circular muscle layer of the esophagus, while the longitudinal layer retains its normal thickness. Additional studies have reported decreased levels of neuronal vasoactive intestinal polypeptide, impairment of postganglionic inhibitory neural pathways, abnormal vagal innervation and eosinophilic infiltration. While the significance of these neural abnormalities in primary (idiopathic) achalasia is unclear, secondary achalasia-like syndromes can occur [i.e. associated with parasitic infiltration (*Trypanosoma cruzi* in Chagas' disease), malignancy, toxins, postvagotomy, infiltrative disorders such as amyloidosis and sarcoidosis, diabetes and following viral infections]. The spectrum of pathophysiologic, clinical and manometric abnormalities seen in classic achalasia may overlap with other primary motor disorders of the esophagus.

Diagnosis

1. Clinical features. Patients most commonly complain of progressive dysphagia to liquids and solids, often over several years. Other symptoms are regurgitation of undigested food, weight loss and coughing or wheezing secondary to aspiration. Occasionally, patients may complain of burning retrosternal chest pain (similar to heartburn), thought to be caused by the fermentation of retained food rather than true gastroesophageal reflux.

2. Radiology and endoscopy. The plain chest X-ray (CXR) is generally normal, but with progression of the disease, a widened mediastinum with an air–fluid level within a dilated esophagus may be seen, especially on the lateral projection. Other findings are absence of a gastric air bubble, or pulmonary infiltrates suggestive of aspiration. A barium swallow may demonstrate a smooth tapering of the distal esophagus (bird's beak) and a dilated or sigmoid esophagus with advanced disease. Absence of peristalis in the body of the esophagus and failure of the LES to relax, may be reported by the radiologist, and are best appreciated by video radiography or radionuclide transit study. The following endoscopic observations may also suggest achalasia: a dilated esophageal body containing a disproportionate amount of food residue (despite fasting for the study), and failure of the esophagogastric junction to open spontaneously with repeated air insufflation (subtle). Both endoscopic and radiologic contrast studies are used to exclude associated foregut malignancy.

3. Esophageal function studies. A definitive diagnosis may be established by esophageal manometry, demonstrating incomplete relaxation of the LES with swallowing and ineffective peristalsis (ultimately aperistalsis) of the body of the esophagus. A hypertensive LES is seen in about half of all patients studied. A variant of classic achalasia which is characterized by high-amplitude, nonperistaltic contractions in the body of the esophagus, is termed vigorous achalasia (see below). Use of ambulatory 24-hour pH studies to document objective acid reflux is often unhelpful because of an abnormally low pH presumed to result from esophageal stasis.

Management

As with all functional disorders of the esophagus, it is essential to establish a precise diagnosis if management is to be successful. The treatment of achalasia is essentially palliative and is directed at relieving obstructive symptoms caused by dysfunction of the LES. The 'trade off' is the potential for developing iatrogenic gastroesophageal reflux.

1. Pneumatic dilation. Mechanical disruption of smooth muscle fibers, achieved by passing a pneumatic balloon across the LES and inflating it to a high pressure, is expected to be successful in about 70% of cases, and should be considered as first-line therapy. In experienced hands, complications of this procedure (i.e. esophageal perforation, gastroesophageal reflux) should be minimal. Although repeated dilation has been advocated, patients who fail two dilations should generally be considered for surgical myotomy.

2. Surgical therapy. Esophagocardiomyotomy, surgical transection of the outer longitudinal and inner circular smooth muscle without damaging the submucosa, is reported to give excellent long-term results (i.e. palliation) in 80–90% of patients with achalasia. Originally described by Heller as an anterior and posterior myotomy the procedure has been modified to a single anterior or lateral myotomy, achieved using an abdominal or thoracic approach. Several controversies persist, principally related to the extent (proximal and distal) of the myotomy, and whether an anti-reflux procedure is needed routinely. The latter should be performed selectively, especially if the distal extent of the myotomy is extended only a limited distance onto the stomach. Excellent early results have recently been achieved using minimally invasive surgical approaches (i.e. laparoscopic or thoracoscopic myotomy). Esophageal resection and reconstruction should be considered in patients who have failed esophageal myotomy (or re-myotomy), or who have an end-stage megaesophagus.

3. Medical therapy. Several pharmacologic agents (i.e. calcium-channel blockers, nitrates, β-agonists) have been used in an attempt to relax the LES, often without clinically significant long-term benefit. Recent attempts have utilized endoscopically injected botulinum toxin. Early results (12–18 months) appear to be comparable with pneumatic dilation, especially in older patients. The sub-group of patients with vigorous achalasia may benefit from this approach.

Vigorous achalasia

In this sub-group of patients with achalasia, chest pain is the predominant symptom. Esophageal manometry often shows high amplitude, nonperistaltic contractions in response to swallowing, in addition to failure of LES relaxation. Treatment is aimed not only at palliating obstructive symptoms, but also at relieving esophageal spasm by extending the myotomy proximally (often to the level of the aortic arch), to include the high-amplitude region of the esophagus as defined manometrically.

Association with malignancy

The association between achalasia and the development of esophageal malignancy is controversial. Prolonged mucosal exposure to dietary carcinogens from esophageal stasis is thought to be a predisposing factor in the development of squamous cell carcinoma. This appears to be relatively uncommon and guidelines for endoscopic surveillance have not been proposed.

Further reading

Csendes A, Braghetto I, Henriquez A, Cortes C. Late results of a prospective randomized study comparing forceful dilation and esophagomyotomy in patients with achalasia. *Gut*, 1989; **30:** 299.

Ellis FH, Watkins E, Gibb, Heatley GJ. Ten to 20-year clinical results after short esophagomyotomy without an antireflux procedure (modified Heller operation) for esophageal achalasia. *European Journal of Cardiothoracic Surgery*, 1992; **6:** 86.

Ferguson MK. Achalasia: current evaluation and therapy. *Annals of Thoracic Surgery*, 1991; **52:** 336.

Graham AJ, Finley RJ, Worsley DF, Dong SR, Clifton JC, Storseth C. Laparoscopic esophageal myotomy and anterior partial fundoplication for the treatment of achalasia. *Annals of Thoracic Surgery*, 1997; **64:** 785.

Orringer MB, Sterling MC. Esophageal resection for achalasia: indications and results. *Annals of Thoracic Surgery*, 1989; **47:** 340.

Pellegrini CA, Leichter R, Patti M, Somberg K. Thoracoscopic esophageal myotomy in the treatment of achalasia. *Annals of Thoracic Surgery*, 1993; **56:** 680.

Related topics of interest

ADULT RESPIRATORY DISTRESS SYNDROME

Fang Gao, Ziv Gamliel

Adult respiratory distress syndrome (ARDS) is a constellation of clinical, radiologic and physiologic abnormalities, characterized by failure of gas exchange leading to hypoxemia, due to pulmonary inflammation and increased capillary permeability.

Etiology

- Sepsis.
- Direct lung contusion/trauma.
- Aspiration of gastric contents.
- Hemorrhagic shock/multiple blood transfusions.
- Multiple organ dysfunction syndrome.
- Pancreatitis.
- Cardiopulmonary bypass.

Pathophysiology

Likely to be a complex series of interrelated events and pathways, activated in response to numerous diverse predisposing factors, resulting in a permeability defect of the pulmonary endothelium. In septic ARDS, macrophages in the pulmonary endothelium, activated by bacteria, generate a biologic cascade releasing cytokines (i.e. tumor necrosis factor, interleukins, platelet activating factors), which cause chemotaxis of neutrophils. Damage to capillary endothelial and type I alveolar cells (mediated by the release of oxygen free radicals) results in increased capillary permeability and flooding of the alveoli with protein-rich fluid. Accumulation of further cellular debris results in the development of hyaline membranes and pulmonary fibrosis after 7–10 days. In nonseptic ARDS it is not clear what triggers the release of cytokines.

Diagnosis

The usual clinical picture is that of rapid onset of hypoxemia, usually within 72 hours of a defined predisposing event. CXR shows bilateral, diffuse, alveolar infiltrates with interstitial edema. Additional diagnostic criteria include:.

- Oxygenation defect defined by a PaO_2/FiO_2 ratio <200 mmHg (27 kPa) regardless of the level of positive end expiratory pressure (PEEP).
- Noncardiogenic pulmonary edema: no clinical evidence of cardiac failure and normal pulmonary capillary wedge pressure (<18 mmHg).

Management

As no specific therapy exists to modulate the sequence of events leading to ARDS, current treatment of this condition is supportive. The objective of pulmonary support is to permit adequate oxygen uptake by the pulmonary capillaries, with minimal barotrauma from mechanical ventilation. Underlying risk factors should be treated.

1. *Monitoring*
   - Patients should be closely monitored in a special unit (i.e. intensive care or high-dependency unit) once the disease is suspected.
   - Clinical observations include heart rate, blood pressure, respiratory rate and temperature.
   - Daily fluid balance, hourly urine output, central venous pressure (CVP) and pulmonary capillary wedge pressure (PCWP) should be used to guide fluid management. Renal function, acid–base balance, electrolyte and nutritional status are assessed.
   - Pulse oximetry, arterial blood gas analysis and CXR are used to monitor the severity of the disease.

2. *Non-ventilatory management*
   - Underlying risk factors are treated.
   - Improve oxygen delivery by increasing the FiO_2, cardiac output (inotropes), or by increasing hemoglobin levels (if necessary).
   - Cardiac output and hemodynamic stability are maintained using the lowest possible CVP or PCWP.
   - Enteral feeding should be started early.
   - Patient positioning may improve gas exchange. This includes kinetic therapy using special rotational beds for periods of 4–8 hours.
   - Inhaled nitric oxide or prostacyclin may improve gas exchange in up to 50% of patients.
   - Extracorporeal membrane oxygenation (ECMO) has not been conclusively proven to improve survival of patients with ARDS and remains investigational.

3. *Ventilatory management*
   - In general, the target for oxygenation is an SaO_2 of >90% or a value for the PaO_2 of >60 mmHg (8 kPa). However, in severe ARDS, lesser values may be accepted provided that acid–base status is maintained and there is no evidence of cerebral edema.
   - Continuous positive airway pressure (CPAP) can be used to improve functional residual capacity in mild disease.
   - PEEP at levels of 10–15 cmH_2O, prevents end-expiratory collapse of alveoli opened during the previous inspiratory cycle. High PEEP can cause barotrauma and hemodynamic instability. The current European view favors the use of higher FiO_2 (up to 1.0), while the North American approach is to keep the FiO_2 <0.6, but to maintain SaO_2 with a higher level of PEEP.
   - The technique of pressure-controlled, inverse inspiratory–expiratory ratio with inspiratory peak pressure <40 cmH_2O

and V_T <10 ml/kg has been shown to provide good gas exchange with hemodynamic stability. Adequate sedation (or paralysis) is often required.
- High-frequency jet ventilation can be used to minimize high airway pressures.

Prognosis

Depends in part on the underlying insult, the presence of other organ dysfunction, age and general health of the patient. Single organ ARDS carries a mortality of 30–50%. Septic ARDS has a higher mortality than nonseptic ARDS. Irreversible respiratory failure, multiorgan failure and sepsis account for most deaths. In patients recovering from ARDS, improvement in lung function may continue for several years.

Further reading

Asbaugh DG, Bigelow DB, Petty TL. Acute respiratory distress in adults. *Lancet*, 1967; **2:** 319.

Brett SJ, Evans TW. Acute lung injury/ARDS. In: Goldhill DR, Withington PS, eds. *Textbook of Intensive Care*. London: Chapman Hall Medical, 1997; 370.

Marini JJ. New approaches to ventilatory management of the adult respiratory distress syndrome. *Journal of Critical Care*, 1992; **7:** 256.

Todd TR, Ralph-Edwards AC. Adult respiratory distress syndrome. In: Pearson FG, Deslauriers J, Ginsberg RJ, Hiebert CA, McKneally MF, Urschel HC, eds. *Thoracic Surgery*. New York: Churchill Livingstone, 1995; 1601.

Related topics of interest

ANESTHESIA FOR THORACIC SURGERY

Fang Gao, Ziv Gamliel

Advances in anesthetic management, associated with increasing complexity of noncardiac thoracic procedures, have resulted in the evolution of the sub-specialty of thoracic anesthesia. It remains essential that the surgeon and anesthetist communicate pre-, intra- and postoperatively, to ensure optimal management of the thoracic patient.

Anesthetic aims
- Maintenance of a clear airway.
- Hemodynamic stability.
- Immediate return to spontaneous breathing after surgery.
- Adequate postoperative analgesia.

Preoperative management

1. Preoperative assessment. See related topic, p. 212.

2. Premedication. Regular cardiovascular and respiratory medications should be taken as usual, but oral hypoglycemic drugs should be omitted. Sedative premedicants should be avoided in patients with poor respiratory reserve. If spinal blocks are planned, anticoagulants should be discontinued.

Intraoperative management

1. Monitoring. Basic monitoring (for all procedures) includes: electrocardiogram (EKG), pulse oximeter, noninvasive blood pressure, end-tidal CO_2 and O_2 analyzer. Additional monitoring (for major thoracic procedures) consists of:

- Arterial cannulation for continuous beat-by-beat direct arterial pressure monitoring and blood-gas sampling.
- Central venous line, for rapid transfusion, infusion of drugs and continuous measurement of right-sided cardiac-filling pressure.
- Pulmonary artery catheters are used infrequently since it is difficult to interpret measurements during one-lung ventilation (OLV) in a lateral position. Transesophageal echocardiography and Doppler have been used to monitor left-sided cardiac function.
- Temperature and urine output.

2. Position
- Lateral decubitus for the majority of intrathoracic procedures.
- Supine for median sternotomy and abdominal approaches.
- Prone, rarely used today.
- Sitting, for postoperative recovery, especially for patients with poor pulmonary reserve.

3. Lung separation. Indicated to improve surgical exposure, to limit soiling of the contralateral lung by blood or pus, and to control ventilation of the contralateral lung without an air leak from alveolar bullae, bronchial or tracheal rupture.

- Double-lumen endotracheal tubes (DLTs) are commonly used for lung separation. DLTs provide independent access to either lung, allowing for two- or one-lung ventilation and suction. Right-sided tubes also incorporate a ventilation slot in the bronchial cuff to provide ventilation to the upper lobe bronchus. Selection of left- or right-sided DLTs:

(a) Intubating the non-operative bronchus allows for unimpeded bronchial surgery, avoiding endobronchial lesions. Technical difficulty in positioning the tube may limit this approach, although a flexible fiberoptic bronchoscope may be useful.

(b) Routine intubation of the left mainstem bronchus eliminates many of the difficulties associated with right-sided tubes and is applicable for all pulmonary resections. Withdrawal of the tube into the trachea during left pneumonectomy may result in the spread of secretions into the contralateral (right) lung.

DLTs are available in disposable and nondisposable forms. Sizes ranging from 39 to 41 F are usually suitable for adult males, 35 to 37 F for females.

- Endobronchial blockers combined with a single lumen endotracheal tube require positioning under bronchoscopic guidance. Advantages are effective exclusion of a lung (or lobe) with massive hemoptysis, with ability to suction the ventilated nonbleeding airway; and ease of postoperative ventilation by withdrawal of the blocker. Disadvantages include a high failure rate of separation (especially on positioning the patient or by surgical manipulation of the lung) and relatively slow lung deflation.

4. One-lung ventilation. During two-lung ventilation, in a lateral decubitus position, ventilation is preferentially diverted to the nondependent lung and perfusion is directed to the dependent lung. This V/Q mismatch is partially reversed when only the dependent lung is ventilated. The unventilated lung will still be perfused to some extent, thus creating a new intrapulmonary shunt. Perfusion to the unventilated lung is limited by hypoxic pulmonary vasoconstriction. This may be reduced by decreased cardiac output, vasodilators and inhalational anesthetic agents, resulting in an increased shunt, which is usually greater in healthy lungs.

Management of one-lung ventilation includes:

- Maintenance of V_T (10 ml/kg) and respiratory rate as for two-lung ventilation.

- 100% O_2.
- Add PEEP to the dependent ventilated lung (5–10 cmH$_2$O).
- Add CPAP to the nonventilated lung.
- Intermittent re-inflation of the nonventilated lung with 100% O_2.
- Clamp the pulmonary artery to the nonventilated lung.
- Additional measures to minimize hypoxemia include avoidance of kinking or malposition of the endotracheal tube or circuit, suctioning secretions, treating broncho-spasm or pneumothorax.

Postoperative management

- Suction and re-inflate nonventilated lung at the end of OLV.
- Return to spontaneous breathing and early extubation.
- Adequate analgesia and chest physiotherapy.
- Monitor in a high-dependency or intensive care unit.

Airway management in selected cases

1. Common features. Awake intubation using a flexible fiberoptic bronchoscope should be considered. Elective post-operative ventilation may be required and appropiate position-ing of the patient is essential.

2. Superior vena cava syndrome. In this syndrome the degree of edema of the upper airway may be comparable with the external appearance. It is important that a sitting position is adopted pre-, intra- and postoperatively. Ventilation with a laryngeal mask has been used successfully to avoid airway intubation for cervical mediastinoscopy.

3. Bronchopleural fistula. In cases of bronchopleural fistula a chest drain should be kept in place until the chest is opened. The patient should breathe spontaneously both before place-ment and after removal of the endotracheal tube. Before intubation, the diseased-side should be positioned down.

4. Tracheoesophageal fistula. In such cases the level and size of the fistula has to be identified. For proximal airway fistulae (to mid-trachea), a single-lumen tube should be used, whereas for distal tracheal fistulae, a carefully positioned double-lumen tube is used.

Further reading

Benumof JL. *Anesthesia for Thoracic Surgery*. Philadelphia: WB Saunders, 1987.

Horlocker TT, Wedel DJ, Schlichting JL. Postoperative epidural analgesia and oral anticoagu-lant therapy. *Anesthesia and Analgesia*, 1994; **79**: 89.

Slinger PD. Fibreoptic bronchoscopic positioning of double-lumen tubes. *Journal of Cardio-thoracic Anesthesia*, 1989; **3**: 486.

Related topics of interest

ANTI-REFLUX SURGERY

Donna E. Maziak, F. Griff Pearson

Although gastroesophageal reflux disease (GERD) is a common condition, relatively few patients will ultimately require anti-reflux surgery. Surgical approaches to correct GERD and its complications have evolved significantly over the past 40 years. Initially, surgeons' performed anatomic repairs to restore esophagogastric anatomy and to correct 'hiatus hernia'. With an improved understanding of foregut physiology, functional anti-reflux procedures (i.e. fundoplication) were devised. That many techniques of anti-reflux surgery have been reported, suggests that no single approach is ideal. Furthermore, with the development of new pharmacologic agents and minimally invasive surgery, the indications and frequency of anti-reflux surgery will continue to change. Finally, a successful outcome depends on establishing an accurate diagnosis of GERD and careful selection of patients for surgery.

Indications

There are relatively few absolute indications for anti-reflux surgery, as GERD and its complications are rarely life threatening. As surgery cannot be guaranteed to be 100% effective, and has a small but definite morbidity (and mortality), one should consider different 'thresholds' for advising anti-reflux surgery in the following situations.

1. Failure of maximal medical therapy (high threshold). The selection of patients with uncomplicated GERD, who have persistent symptoms that interfere with their normal lifestyle, is particularly challenging. Such patients should be proven to have objective evidence of GERD, and should have received maximal medical therapy for at least 6 months. Full discussion of the potential complications of surgery is warranted prior to making a final decision regarding surgery.

2. Complications of GERD (low threshold)
- Peptic stricture.
- Ulcerative esophagitis.
- Recurrent aspiration and/or pneumonia.
- Barrett's esophagus (to correct GERD-related symptoms).

Principles of surgery

The aims of surgery are as follows: creation of an intra-abdominal segment of esophagus (if the esophagus is short); the creation of an anti-reflux mechanism (i.e. fundoplication) that allows normal swallowing, belching and vomiting, but prevents pathologic gastroesophageal reflux; and prevention of herniation of the esophagogastric junction (and fundoplication) into the chest.

Operative approaches

1. Route. The esophageal surgeon should be familiar with several surgical approaches to the esophagus and esophagogastric junction:

- Abdominal. This is most effective with a normal length (abdominal) esophagus. Open procedures have now generally been superceded by laparoscopic approaches.
- Thoracic. This is traditionally used for the Belsey Mark IV partial fundoplication, but is excellent when esophageal lengthening (Collis gastroplasty) is required.
- Thoracoabdominal. Most useful for reoperative surgery.
- Laparoscopic. A major advance. Well accepted by patients. Short-term results are encouraging, but the long-term efficacy is still unproven. However, results should be comparable if the indications for anti-reflux surgery, and the technique of fundoplication, remain the same.

2. *Fundoplication.* Experimental and clinical evidence suggest that a total (360°) fundoplication is more effective at restoring lower esophageal sphincter pressure and preventing reflux. However, the precise mechanism of action of a fundoplication is unclear. A fundoplication does not function properly if situated in the chest (probably related to negative intrathoracic pressure). Therefore, it is imperative that the fundoplication be placed within the abdomen.

- 360° (Nissen). May be performed successfully using any approach. Excision of the fat pad at the esophagogastric junction; division of a variable number of short gastric vessels; use of a large bougie (>50 F); and performing a 2-cm fundoplication, utilizing three nonabsorbable sutures incorporating the esophageal wall, increase the success of this procedure.
- 270° (Belsey Mark IV). A transthoracic approach, utilizing two to three rows of horizontal mattress sutures, is used to plicate the gastric fundus around the mobilized esophagus, which is reduced without tension below the diaphragm.
- Partial. Increasingly performed laparoscopically. The Toupet fundoplication involves suturing the posteriorly sited fundus to the right and left crura to create a 180–270° wrap, whereas the Dor repair comprises a 180° anterior wrap.
- Hill gastropexy. Involves suturing fundus to the median arcuate ligament.

3. *Esophageal lengthening.* In the presence of esophageal shortening, Collis described a technique (*Figure 1*) to create a lesser curve gastric tube (neoesophagus) that would permit the creation of a tension-free intra-abdominal fundoplication. A transthoracic approach is preferred, particularly to assess esophageal shortening and to dilate an esophageal stricture under direct vision. A mechanical linear cutting stapler is positioned parallel to a large bougie held against the lesser curve of

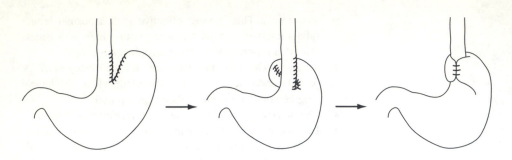

Figure 1. Stages of the total (Collis–Nissen) fundoplication procedure.

the stomach and, starting at the esophagogastric junction, the stapler is fired to create a gastric tube with a diameter similar to the esophagus. The suture line is oversewn and a partial (Collis–Belsey) or total (Collis–Nissen) fundoplication performed around the neoesophagus, which is reduced below the diaphragm. Recent reports suggest efficacy of an 'uncut' gastroplasty.

4. Closure of the crura. This is an integral component of the anti-reflux procedure, to prevent migration of the fundoplication into the mediastinum. Interrupted nonabsorbable sutures should be used to approximate the crura posteriorly, with a bougie in the esophagus, sufficient to accept the tip of a finger.

Choice of anti-reflux procedure

For uncomplicated GERD, without significant esophageal shortening, a transabdominal (laparoscopic) total (Nissen) fundoplication is preferred. In the presence of poor esophageal motor function (assessed by preoperative manometry), a partial fundoplication would be appropiate (laparoscopic or Belsey). With esophageal shortening, a transthoracic approach is preferred. A Collis gastroplasty is combined with a total fundoplication (Nissen) if good motor function is demonstrated, or with a partial fundoplication (Belsey) if motility is shown to be poor.

Specific complications

1. Dysphagia. Related to the extent of fundoplication (i.e. too long, too tight), or the presence of an associated motility disorder.

2. 'Gas bloat' syndrome. Characterized by the inability to belch and postprandial fullness. It is often of multifactorial etiology (vagal nerve injury, aerophagia, delayed gastric emptying, extent of fundoplication, etc.).

3. Technical failures. 'Slipped Nissen', breakdown of the fundoplication, herniation into the mediastinum, esophageal or gastric perforation.

Results

The long-term results of anti-reflux surgery should be considered at 10, 15 and 20 years. The generally quoted results are 85–90% successful (good/excellent results) according to surveyed patients undergoing Nissen fundoplication. For the Belsey technique the results are slightly less successful (post-thoracotomy pain vs. less dysphagia vs. recurrence of reflux symptoms). Initial results of laparoscopic surgery are encouraging, but long-term follow-up is essential.

Further reading

Henderson RD, Henderson RF, Marryatt GV. Surgical management of 100 consecutive esophageal strictures. *Journal of Thoracic and Cardiovascular Surgery*, 1990; **99:** 1.

Jamieson GG, Watson DI, Britten-Jones R, Mitchell PC, Anvani M. Laparoscopic Nissen fundoplication. *Annals of Surgery*, 1994; **220:** 137.

Kaur WKH, Peters JH, DeMeester TR. A tailored approach to antireflux surgery. *Journal of Thoracic and Cardiovascular Surgery*, 1995; **110:** 141.

Little AG. Mechanisms of action of antireflux surgery: theory and fact. *World Journal of Surgery,* 1992; **16:** 320.

Pearson FG, Cooper JD, Patterson GA, Ramirez J, Todd TR. Gastroplasty and fundoplication for complex reflux problems. Long-term results. *Annals of Surgery*, 1987; **206:** 473.

Peters JH, DeMeester TR. Indications, benefits and outcome of laparoscopic Nissen fundoplication. *Digest of Disease*, 1996; **14:** 169.

Related topics of interest

BARRETT'S ESOPHAGUS

Alan G. Casson

There has been considerable recent interest in the columnar epithelium-lined (Barrett's) esophagus, which is believed to result from chronic gastroesophageal reflux disease. The clinical importance of Barrett's esophagus is related to its association with esophageal malignancy, particularly adenocarcinomas, which have increased in incidence rapidly over the past several decades. However, the natural history of this condition is not known with certainty and it remains a controversial entity.

Definition

Several definitions have been proposed. The most satisfactory working definitions require both a histologic and endoscopic diagnosis, as follows.

The classic diagnosis, based entirely on endoscopic findings, requires the squamo-columnar junction to be greater than 3 cm above the anatomic esophagogastric junction (EGJ). This has several limitations: the 3-cm level is empiric, the squamo-columnar junction is often irregular (limiting accurate measurements) and endoscopic detection of the anatomic EGJ (defined as the point where the tubular esophagus joins the saccular stomach) is often imprecise, for example in the presence of a hiatus hernia.

A more recent definition is the histologic finding of specialized columnar epithelium, characterized by intestinal metaplasia, in biopsies taken at any level of the tubular esophagus (determined endoscopically). This definition would be satisfactory to diagnose 'short-segment' Barrett's esophagus (within the distal 3 cm of the esophagus). The principal difficulty with this definition is histopathologic and relates to the definition of metaplasia. Normal distal esophageal columnar epithelium (<3 cm) is cardiac- or fundic-type. Metaplastic epithelium is defined by the presence of goblet cells, containing acid mucins, which stain positively with Alcian blue at pH 2.5.

Epidemiology

- The prevalence of Barrett's esophagus in symptomatic (i.e. heartburn, dyspepsia) patients undergoing endoscopy ranges from 8 to 12%.
- The prevalence in the general (asymptomatic) population is <1%.
- Short-segment Barrett's esophagus may be found in up to 18% of unselected patients undergoing endoscopy for various reasons.
- Although Barrett's esophagus has been diagnosed in infants and children (associated with GERD), the median age of diagnosis is 50 years.
- It is not known with certainty whether the true incidence of Barrett's esophagus is increasing, or whether greater

recognition of this finding has resulted from increased access to esophagoscopy.

Etiology and pathogenesis

Chronic gastroesophageal reflux (and esophagitis) is believed to injure the squamous epithelium lining the esophagus, which usually heals by regeneration of squamous mucosa. Unknown healing mechanisms are responsible for the replacement of squamous epithelium by columnar cells, which proliferate to form an abnormal epithelium. It is believed that replacement can occur rapidly, within 4–6 weeks of the initiating reflux event.

The majority of patients with Barrett's esophagus have some degree of objective esophageal dysfunction, predisposing to reflux. This includes: increased esophageal exposure to refluxed gastric acid, particularly at night-time; increased exposure to refluxed duodenal contents (duodenogastroesophageal reflux); LES dysfunction (i.e. inappropiate relaxation, hypotension); delayed esophageal clearance; and increased gastric-acid secretion. These clinical observations are also supported in experimental models.

Barrett's epithelium has also been reported in patients receiving cytotoxic chemotherapy. Other factors, such as tobacco and alcohol intake, are associated with the development of Barrett's epithelium. The role of *Helicobacter pylori* infection is unknown.

To date the natural history of Barrett's esophagus, its potential for regression, stabilization or progression, is not known.

Association with esophageal malignancy

It is well established that Barrett's esophagus predisposes to esophageal cancer, particularly adenocarcinomas. However, it may also be a risk factor for esophageal squamous-cell carcinoma. The magnitude of the cancer risk is unknown and estimates are controversial as they are based on relatively few patient numbers and short follow-up. Currently, the incidence of developing a Barrett's adenocarcinoma (per patient year) ranges from 1 in 52 to 1 in 175.

Dysplasia, particularly high-grade dysplasia, in Barrett's esophagus is currently the only clinically relevant factor that identifies patients at increased risk for the development of esophageal cancer. Dysplasia is recognized histologically, and may be defined as neoplastic epithelium confined within the epithelial surface within which it arose. In low-grade dysplasia, crypt architecture tends to be preserved with minimal distortion and cells with atypical hyperchromatic nuclei are limited to the basal half of the crypts. In high-grade dysplasia, the nuclei are larger, more hyperchromatic, have irregular nuclear membranes and have lost their polarity. Architecturally, there appears to be more crypt distortion, and differentiation of high-grade dysplasia from invasive carcinoma (where cells have penetrated the basement membrane to infiltrate the lamina propia) may be very difficult. Although the finding of high-grade dysplasia in Barrett's esophagus is frequently (about 40–50%) associated with adenocarcinoma, this is not inevitable.

It is believed that esophageal adenocarcinomas develop as a multistep process, characterized histologically as a sequentially progressive dysplasia to carcinoma sequence. Recent studies suggest that accumulation of molecular genetic alterations underlies the process of malignant transformation, although the relative importance of individual genetic lesions and the sequence of genetic events leading to esophageal tumor development, is yet to be determined.

Diagnosis

1. Clinical presentation. The majority of patients with Barrett's esophagus are diagnosed incidentally during investigation of symptoms related to associated GERD.

2. Radiology. Contrast studies of the esophagus often do not show sufficient mucosal detail to establish the diagnosis of Barrett's mucosa with certainty. However, reflux-related findings (i.e. ulceration, strictures) may be detected.

3. Endoscopy and biopsy. The endoscopic appearance of long-segment Barrett's mucosa is typical, and is based on measurement (>3 cm) and appearance (a deeper pink color compared with pale squamous mucosa). Biopsy is essential to confirm the diagnosis, especially of short-segment Barrett's esophagus. The technique of biopsy is important, and should include use of large-cup forceps; multiple biopsies are taken systematically at 2-cm intervals along columnar-lined esophagus, incorporating the esophagogastric junction and proximal squamous epithelium. Abnormal mucosal lesions should be biopsied to exclude carcinoma. Endoscopic application of vital stains (i.e. Lugol's iodine, toluidine blue) may improve recognition of columnar mucosa and possibly increase the sensitivity of the endoscopic biopsy technique. However, this is not widely used in clinical practice.

Management

The goal of treatment of Barrett's esophagus is the control of associated symptoms of GERD and the prevention of reflux-related complications (i.e. stricture). This is achieved by medical and surgical anti-reflux therapy (see related topics of interest).

However, neither medical nor surgical therapy have consistently been shown to alter the length of the columnar-lined esophagus, nor have they proved to be effective in reducing the risk of malignant degeneration.

Screening patients with Barrett's esophagus (including patients who have been treated medically or who have undergone anti-reflux surgery) remains controversial. Recent studies suggest that endoscopic surveillance can detect early stage adenocarcinomas in Barrett's esophagus, and that early detection and surgical resection may decrease mortality rates from esophageal cancer in these patients.

Current recommendations for endoscopic surveillance are as follows.

1. *Barrett's esophagus without dysplasia.* Screening every 18–24 months.

2. *Low-grade dysplasia.* Re-biopsy after 6–12 weeks of medical anti-reflux therapy is recommended, to exclude the possibility that inflammatory change was interpreted as low-grade dysplasia. If low-grade dysplasia is confirmed, screening every 6–12 months is recommended.

3. *High-grade dysplasia.* Re-biopsy to confirm the diagnosis. Options include:

- Surgical resection. Recommended treatment, assuming minimal operative risk. Unsuspected (undiagnosed) carcinoma is encountered in up to 50% of resected specimens.
- Ongoing surveillance. Probably should be reserved for higher risk surgical patients. The frequency of surveillance is also not known.
- Mucosal ablation therapy, using electrocoagulation, laser, argon beam, photodynamic therapy or surgical mucosectomy, is currently under evaluation.

4. *Invasive adenocarcinoma.* Management of histologically proven invasive carcinoma is the same as for any esophageal adenocarcinoma (see 'Esophageal cancer: etiology and pathology', p. 88). Improved screening to identify high-risk patients may, in future, involve assessment of molecular genetic markers, or flow-cytometry.

Further reading

Bremner CG, DeMeester TR. Proceedings from an international conference on ablation therapy for Barrett's mucosa. *Diseases of the Esophagus*, 1998; **11:** 1.

DeMeester TR. Barrett's esophagus. *Surgery*, 1993; **113:** 239.

Dent J, Bremner CG, Collen MJ, Haggitt RC, Spechler SJ. Barrett's esophagus. *Journal of Gastrology and Hepatology*, 1991; **6:** 1.

Schneider PM, Casson AG, Roth JA. Malignant degeneration of Barrett's esophagus. *Diseases of the Esophagus*, 1995; **8:** 99.

Stein HJ, Hoeft S, Korn O, Siewert JR. Gastroduodenal function in Barrett's esophagus. *Diseases of the Esophagus*, 1995; **8:** 205.

Streitz JM. Barrett's esophagus and esophageal cancer. *Chest Surgery Clinics of North America*, 1994; **4:** 227.

Related topics of interest

BENIGN ESOPHAGEAL TUMORS

Simon Pickard, Renee Kennedy

Benign tumors of the esophagus are rare. They may arise from any layer of the esophageal wall and at any level. Most are asymptomatic, but intermittent dysphagia or other vague swallowing changes are occasionally reported.

Classification (by esophageal layer of origin)

1. Mucosa
- Epithelium. Squamous cell papilloma, adenoma or adenomatous hyperplasia.
- Lamina propia. Mucus retention cyst, fibrovascular polyp, inflammatory pseudotumor.
- Muscularis mucosae. Leiomyoma.

2. Submucosa
- Mucous gland. Mucus retention cyst, adenoma.
- Connective tissue. Fibrovascular polyp.
- Blood vessels. Hemangioma.
- Neural tissue. Neurilemmoma, granular cell tumor.

3. Muscularis propia
- Striated muscle. Rhabdomyoma.
- Smooth muscle. Leiomyoma.
- Neural tissue. Neurofibroma, neurilemmoma, granular cell tumor.

4. Adventitia
- Connective tissue. Fibroma.
- Neural tissue. Neurilemmoma.

Management

The majority of benign esophageal tumors are identified by barium-swallow examination, or at the time of endoscopy. As a tissue diagnosis is essential to exclude a malignant esophageal tumor, biopsy of all esophageal lesions should be performed. However, care should be taken if the lesion is intramural with an intact mucosa. Occasionally endoscopic excision of pedunculated benign tumors may be performed. Additional noninvasive investigations, including computed tomography (CT) scanning and endoscopic ultrasound may be helpful in suggesting a benign diagnosis, or planning needle biopsy or surgical approaches. Surgery is performed to obtain a definitive diagnosis and for symptomatic tumors. Local excision of small tumors may be performed by thoracotomy or video-assisted thoracoscopic surgery (VATS). Esophageal resection and reconstruction may be required for larger lesions.

Specific benign esophageal lesions

1. Leiomyoma/leiomyosarcoma. Characteristically present as a slow-growing, solitary lesion, causing slit-like compression of the esophageal lumen. Esophageal obstruction is uncommon unless the lesion is greater than 5 cm in diameter, or has grown circumferentially to encase the esophagus. These tumors have a typical radiologic appearance (barium contrast) and endoscopically, the overlying esophageal mucosa is intact. Leiomyomas are benign tumors of smooth muscle, comprising well-differentiated, elongated fusiform cells with eosinophilic cytoplasm. It is unlikely that they progress to malignancy. Differentiation from a leiomyosarcoma may be difficult, although these malignant tumors will have increased cellularity, mitoses, nuclear atypia and necrosis. Tumors should be removed if symptoms develop, if rapid growth occurs or to establish a definite diagnosis. Surgical removal of leiomyomas may be performed using VATS or by thoracotomy. The esophageal muscle is opened longitudinally and the tumor enucleated. Care is taken not to damage the esophageal mucosa.

2. Granular cell tumor. The cell of origin of these unusual tumors is believed to be a perineural (Schwann) cell. Esophagoscopy reveals a firm, sessile, polypoid nodule, with intact mucosa. Lesions smaller than 2 cm should be observed only. Larger lesions, those showing rapid growth or if symptomatic, should be treated by local surgical excision. The submucosal origin of these tumors precludes endoscopic removal.

3. Fibrovascular polyp. Occur in older males, as solitary pedunculated lesions, typically originating in the upper esophagus. With growth, these tumors extend into the esophageal lumen where they may become quite large. Most are asymptomatic, but they can produce esophageal obstruction (ie. dysphagia), airway obstruction (if regurgitated), or bleed (from mucosal ulceration). Resection (endoscopic or thoracotomy) is recommended.

4. Squamous cell papilloma. May be related to human papilloma virus infection. Endoscopic appearance is typical (firm, multilobulated, wart-like appearance), but biopsy is essential to exclude verrucous squamous-cell carcinoma. Endoscopic removal of obstructing lesions is usually successful, but occasionally thoracotomy and local excision is required.

5. Adenoma. Visualized endoscopically as a polypoid mass developing within a columnar epithelium-lined esophagus. Biopsies should be evaluated carefully to determine the degree of dysplastic change. Metaplasia and low-grade dysplasia warrant endoscopic surveillance. High-grade dysplasia (suggesting an increased risk of malignancy) or the presence of invasive adenocarcinoma, should be managed by esophageal resection and reconstruction.

Further reading

Shamji F, Todd TRJ. Benign tumors. In: Pearson FG, Deslauriers J, Ginsberg RJ, Hiebert CA, McKneally MF, Urschel HC, eds. *Esophageal Surgery*. New York: Churchill Livingstone, 1995; 519.

Related topics of interest

BENIGN LUNG TUMORS

Simon Pickard, Alan G. Casson

These tumors are rare, but with the advent of minimally invasive surgical techniques, are being referred to thoracic surgeons for resection with increasing frequency. Classification of these tumors has been controversial, as the cell of origin and natural history of many of these tumors are largely unknown.

Classification (by origin, with approximate percentage)

1. *Epithelial*
   - Polyps.
   - Papilloma.
   - Bronchial mucous gland adenoma (1%).

2. *Mesodermal*
   - Chrondroma.
   - Fibroma (12%).
   - Granular cell tumor (schwannoma).
   - Lipoma (1.5%).
   - Leiomyoma (1.5%).
   - Sclerosing hemangioma.
   - Hemangiopericytoma.

3. *Unknown*
   - Hamartoma (77%).
   - Clear cell tumor (sugar tumor).

4. *Others*
   - Plasma cell granuloma.
   - Germ cell tumors (teratoma).
   - Xanthoma and inflammatory pseudotumors (5%).
   - Amyloid.
   - Mucosa-associated lymphoid tumors (pseudolymphoma).
   - Mixed tumors (1%).

Management

The majority of benign tumors are identified as incidental findings on CXR, as a solitary lung nodule, which is asymptomatic. Review of previous films is essential. CT scanning and needle biopsy may occasionally suggest a benign diagnosis, but a definitive tissue diagnosis can only be made following excision, which is also curative. Recent advances in minimally invasive surgery (video-assisted thoracoscopic surgery, VATS) have lowered the threshold for early referral and surgical excision. Occasionally benign tumors may present with atelectasis and airway obstruction, suggesting an endobronchial origin. In this situation, rigid bronchoscopy will be diagnostic and therapeutic.

Specific benign tumors

1. Hamartoma. The most common benign lung tumor, seen at all ages with a slight male predominance. Histologically, it comprises an abnormal collection of normal lung tissue components (i.e. cartilage, fat, glands). Radiographically, hamartomas appear as well-circumscribed single nodules, generally up to 2 cm in size, which may be located in any part of the lung. CT scanning may show calcification and fat in up to half of all lesions. Tumors are generally slow growing, and may therefore be followed radiographically if excision is not performed.

2. Lipoma. Predominantly arising from submucosal fat between the cartilaginous rings of the bronchus. Most present with endobronchial symptoms (i.e. airway obstruction, atelectasis etc.), and may be treated by bronchoscopic excision.

3. Sclerosing hemangioma. Occurs most frequently in middle-aged women as a solitary, well-circumscribed nodule which may be partially calcified. Four major histologic patterns are reported: solid, papillary, vascular and sclerotic. The finding of multiple tumors suggests a malignant variant of this tumor.

4. Hemangiopericytoma. This tumor, derived from capillary pericytes, is characterized by its vascularity and surrounding spindle-shaped cells (suggesting a sarcoma). It may behave as a benign or malignant tumor and should therefore be excised.

Further reading

Kaiser LR, Bavaria JE. Benign lung tumors. In: Pearson FG, Deslauriers J, Ginsberg RJ, Hiebert CA, McKneally MF, Urschel HC, eds. *Thoracic Surgery*. New York: Churchill Livingstone, 1995; 613.

Related topics of interest

BRONCHOPLASTIC (SLEEVE) PROCEDURES

Sean Grondin, Michael R. Johnston

Bronchoplastic or sleeve resection is an alternative to pneumonectomy. It is a lung-sparing procedure, typically used to resect proximal endobronchial lesions (at or adjacent to the carina) in an effort to preserve more distal, uninvolved lung parenchyma. Occasionally, resection and reanastomosis of the pulmonary artery, as well as the bronchus, may be necessary and such procedures may be technically challenging. Results of bronchoplastic procedures in selected patients are comparable with standard pulmonary resection.

Indications

- Low-grade endobronchial malignant tumors of the major airways, such as typical carcinoid, mucoepidermoid and adenoid cystic carcinomas.
- Non-small cell lung cancer (NSCLC) with proximal bronchial extention such that lobectomy would result in tumor at the resection margin. Optimal results are, however, obtained in patients without lymph-node metastases.
- Benign lesions, such as post-traumatic or inflammatory stricture.
- In a patient that cannot tolerate a more extensive resection (i.e. pneumonectomy) because of limited pulmonary function.

Technique

Applicable to anatomically suitable lesions of either main bronchus or any of the five major lobar bronchi. May include: a sleeve lobectomy, comprising excision of a lobe with the associated lobar bronchus and involving anastomosis of the distal bronchial tree to the proximal airway; bronchial sleeve resection, comprising resection of either mainstem bronchus, with anastomosis of the distal airway to the carina or lower trachea; or sleeve pneumonectomy, comprising resection of the carina with pneumonectomy and anastomosis of the contralateral distal bronchus to the distal trachea.

1. Preoperative evaluation
- Bronchoscopy, to define the anatomic location of the lesion, with biopsy.
- Radiographic studies, including linear tomography (where available), or CT scanning (and coronal reconstruction).
- Mediastinoscopy, to exclude mediastinal lymph-node metastases from NSCLC, should be performed on the day of the planned bronchoplasty to facilitate mobilization of the tracheobronchial tree and avoid adhesions.
- General considerations for general anesthesia and pulmonary resection.

2. Anesthetic. Selective intubation of the distal airway, either by advancing the endotracheal tube or by direct placement across the operative field, will usually be necessary. However, high-frequency jet ventilation may also be used successfully.

3. Surgery. Surgical principles include precise approximation of the airways, minimal mucosal handling, maintenance of the bronchial collateral circulation by preserving peribronchial tissues and utilization of a tension-free anastomosis. This usually requires some degree of mobilization of the tracheobronchial tree and, at minimum, division of the inferior pulmonary ligament. Incision of the pericardium (infrahilar or circumferential release as required) or reimplantation of the inferior pulmonary vein are described, but are rarely necessary.

Coverage of the anastomosis with an intercostal muscle flap, pericardium, pleura or omentum to minimize dehiscence and subsequent formation of a bronchopleural fistula. This is especially important if radiation therapy is utilized pre- or postoperatively.

Several anastomotic techniques are reported, including telescoping the distal bronchus into the proximal airway. Utilization of fine, interrupted, absorbable sutures, with knots placed externally, appears to reduce granuloma and stricture formation.

Mobilization, preservation and orientation of associated arterial and venous structures. Occasionally, sleeve vascular resection is also necessary.

Complications

- Leak or dehiscence of the bronchial anastomosis (bronchopleural fistula) is seen in up to 3% of sleeve lobectomies and up to 10% of sleeve pneumonectomies.
- Retained secretions and pneumonia in lung distal to the anastomosis. Prevention of this postoperative complication requires early mobilization, chest physiotherapy and frequent bronchoscopy, expediently performed at the bedside using local anesthesia only, to aspirate secretions from the distal airway.
- Torsion, narrowing or stenosis of the bronchial anastomosis.
- Bronchovascular fistula, especially with combined bronchial and arterial sleeve resections, is usually fatal.
- Empyema, pulmonary embolus, respiratory failure, cardiac dysrhythmias, etc.

Results

The mortality rate (30-day) for all bronchoplastic procedures is 8%, with rates for sleeve lobectomy of 5% and sleeve pneumonectomy 20–25%. Causes of death are respiratory failure (ARDS, pulmonary edema, pneumonia), myocardial infarction (and dysrhythmias), pulmonary embolus and bronchial complications. Long-term functional results and exercise tolerance are superior to pneumonectomy. Overall and disease-free survival rates depend on the primary pathology. For NSCLC, bronchoplastic procedures are comparable with standard resections, with complete resection (negative resection margins) and absence of regional lymph node metastases (N0) being the best predictors of long-term survival.

Further reading

Bueno R, Wain JC, Wright CD. Bronchoplasty in the management of low-grade airway malignancies and benign bronchial stenoses. *Annals of Thoracic Surgery*, 1996; **62:** 824.
Gaissert HA, Mathisen DJ, Moncure AC. Survival and function after sleeve lobectomy for lung cancer. *Journal of Thoracic and Cardiovascular Surgery*, 1996; **111:** 948.
Tedder M, Anstadt MP, Tedder SD, Lowe JE. Current morbidity, mortality and survival after bronchoplastic procedures for malignancy. *Annals of Thoracic Surgery*, 1992; **54:** 387.

Related topics of interest

BRONCHOPLEURAL FISTULA

Alan G. Casson

Bronchopleural fistulae are generally associated with an infected pleural space (i.e. empyema), and may result in persistent sepsis, failure of re-expansion of the ipsilateral lung and contamination of the contralateral lung. Management and prognosis depend on the etiology of the fistula, its anatomic location (i.e. central airway vs. peripheral alveolar leakage) and its associated complications.

Etiology

1. Postoperative. Most bronchopleural fistulae (of varying severity) occur following pulmonary resection (i.e. pneumonectomy, lobectomy, sleeve resections), and are reported in up to 3% of all patients. The following factors are of importance:

- Surgical technique. Appropiate technical closure of the bronchus or lung tissue.
- Adjuvant therapies. Pre- or postoperative chemoradiotherapy.
- Infection. Endobronchial bacterial or tuberculous infections, drug-resistant organisms.
- Associated illness. Chronic nutritional deficiency, systemic steroid therapy.
- Recurrent tumor.

2. Spontaneous fistula. May occur in association with:

- Pneumonia; bacterial, or associated with AIDS.
- Lung abscess.
- Tuberculosis.
- Spontaneous pneumothorax; particularly where associated with chronic obstructive lung disease.

3. Traumatic. Following penetrating or blunt airway injury.

Diagnosis

Suspect a bronchopleural fistula associated with an empyema. May be diagnosed radiographically by an air/fluid level. A persistent air leak following chest tube insertion, failure of the ipsilateral lung to re-expand, persistent cough and sputum production (often blood tinged) in certain positions, recurrent contralateral pneumonias are often found to some degree. Bronchoscopy, CT scanning and radionuclide ventilation scanning may be useful to confirm the diagnosis and etiology of the fistula (i.e. to demonstrate recurrent tumor). *Postpneumonectomy* fistula is a special situation and should always be suspected when a drop in the fluid level (usually to the level of the bronchial stump) is seen on an upright postoperative CXR, or when a patient suddenly develops cough productive of copious salmon-colored fluid.

Management

Depends on the etiology of the fistula, the timing of fistula development (if postoperative), and the severity of co-morbid disease. Initial management often parallels that of the associated empyema. However, selected patients may benefit from definitive surgical closure of the fistula.

1. General. Intravenous fluids and antibiotics, enteral nutrition, chest physiotherapy and supplemental oxygen, as indicated clinically.

2. Chest tube drainage. All pleural collections should be drained early, to control pleural sepsis and permit re-expansion of the underlying lung. Chest drains should be of sufficient diameter (not less than 28 F) and connected to underwater seal drainage. Use of suction is controversial, as it is widely believed that this will cause the fistula to persist. It may also cause clinically significant dyspnoea and oxygen desaturation by decreasing effective tidal volume. However, suction may be applied carefully to the chest drainage system (monitoring the patient clinically), and if tolerated, should be used initially to ensure pleural drainage and expansion of any underlying lung tissue. More than one drain may be used. If this is not tolerated, or the lung does not re-expand fully, suction is discontinued and chest tubes are placed onto underwater seal drainage alone. Long-term drainage may be achieved by converting to an empyema tube or creating a surgical thoracostomy.

3. Surgery. Several surgical approaches to close a bronchopleural fistula are described. The following criteria should be considered predictive of long-term success:

- No recurrent tumor.
- Control of any associated empyema/sepsis.
- Acceptable anesthetic risk.

Peripheral fistulae originating from lung parenchyma will generally seal provided full re-expansion of the remaining lung is achieved. Occasionally thoracotomy and direct suture (buttressed) or mechanical stapling, is required. A pleurectomy (or abrasion) is advised to obliterate the pleural space. Attempts to seal, coagulate or laser lung tissue, particularly using VATS approaches, have generally met with limited long-term success. The most difficult decision is often the timing of surgery.

In general, the use of fibrin sealants (glue) applied to a central (i.e. mainstem or lobar) bronchial fistula through the bronchoscope, has proved disappointing. Thoracotomy with closure of the fistula may be appropiate for selected patients. Direct suture alone is generally inadequate, and the suture line should be reinforced with healthy local tissues (i.e. pericardial or pleural flaps) or a vascular muscle flap. A right thoracotomy may be used to approach either a right or left mainstem bronchus fistula. An associated empyema cavity should also be controlled by interposing muscle (preferred) or thoracoplasty.

Alternatively, a sternotomy may be used (Perelman). In the unusual situation where a bronchopleural fistula persists following lobectomy (especially with recurrent localized tumor), consideration should be given to completion pneumonectomy.

Postpneumonectomy bronchopleural fistula

A high index of suspicion should be maintained throughout the postoperative course. Management depends on the timing of the fistula in relation to surgery.

For patients within the first to second postoperative week: position the operated side down; drain the postpneumonectomy space (open the wound or place a chest tube connected to an underwater seal alone – no suction); oxygen should be used if breathing spontaneously, however, intubation and high-frequency ventilation must be considered if respiratory failure occurs; intravenous (IV) fluids and antibiotics are used as indicated clinically. Bronchoscopy is performed to evaluate the bronchial stump. If this appears to be grossly intact, nonoperative management may be indicated. If the fistula appears large, reoperation is generally required to close the fistula (as described above).

For patients over two weeks postoperatively: the pneumonectomy space should be drained with a chest tube. When stable convert to open drainage (thoracostomy/Eloesser flap) and close the thoracostomy 3–6 months later (Claggett procedure), after the empyema has resolved and the bronchopleural fistula is closed. If the fistula is secondary to tumor recurrence, closure is unlikely.

Further reading

Claggett OT, Geraci JE. A procedure for the management of postpneumonectomy empyema. *Journal of Thoracic and Cardiovascular Surgery*, 1963; **45**: 141.

Eloesser L. An operation for tuberculous empyema. *Surgery, Gynecology and Obstetrics*, 1935; **60**: 1096.

Ginsberg RJ, Pearson FG, Cooper JD. Closure of chronic bronchopleural fistula using a transsternal transpericardial approach. *Annals of Thoracic Surgery*, 1989; **47**: 231.

Miller JI, ed. Empyema, spaces and fistula. *Chest Surgery Clinics of North America*, 1996; **6**: 403.

Pairolero PC, Trastek VF, Allen MS. Empyema and bronchopleural fistula. *Annals of Thoracic Surgery*, 1991; **51**: 157.

Perelman ME, Rymko LP. Management of empyemas: the problems of associated bronchopleural fistulae. In: Deslauriers J, Lacquet LK, eds. *International Trends in General Thoracic Surgery*. St. Louis: CV Mosby, 1990; 301.

York JEL, Lewall DB, Hirji M. Endoscopic diagnosis and treatment of postoperative bronchopleural fistula. *Chest*, 1990; **197**: 1390.

Related topics of interest

BRONCHOSCOPY

Shaf Keshafjee, Hani K. Najm

The bronchoscope is an invaluable instrument to all surgeons dealing with diseases of the respiratory system. In addition to being an essential diagnostic modality, it provides direct therapeutic benefit in several situations. The rigid bronchoscope was introduced in the 1950s and the flexible bronchoscopy in the 1970s. Since then, the indications and techniques for each have evolved. Rigid and flexible bronchoscopy should be considered complementary to each other in their diagnostic and therapeutic applications in the management of thoracic diseases.

Indications for flexible bronchoscopy

1. Diagnostic
- Abnormal radiographic finding.
- Acute inhalation injury.
- Bronchietasis.
- Broncholithiasis.
- Cough.
- Foreign body.
- Hemoptysis.
- Intubation injury.
- Lung abcess.
- Sputum cytology suspicious for cancer.
- Stridor or localized wheezing.
- Thoracic trauma.
- Vocal-cord paralysis.

2. Therapeutic
- Retained secretions or mucus plugs (bronchial toilet).
- Laser therapy.
- Difficult endotracheal intubation.
- Foreign-body removal.
- Lung abscess.
- Brachytherapy.
- Bronchopleual fistula.

Indications for rigid bronchoscopy
- Massive hemoptysis.
- Airway obstruction: diagnostic and therapeutic.
- Foreign body.
- Tumor: endobronchial, extrinsic compression.
- Benign stricture.
- Laser therapy.
- Endobronchial stenting.
- Tracheobronchial toilet.
- Pediatric bronchoscopy.

Contraindications

Contraindications are relative and do not necessarily preclude a carefully performed bronchoscopy. Relative contraindications to flexible bronchoscopy include:

- Bleeding disorders – whether pathologic or anticoagulant induced.
- Hypoxemia and hypercapnia.
- Cardiovascular instability – hypotension, uncontrolled angina, malignant arrhythmia, recent myocardial infarction.
- Severe asthma.
- Patients unable to cooperate with the procedure.

Extra care should be practised in patients with active TB, HIV and hepatitis to avoid possible spread of the organism, and where there is a tracheal obstruction, due to the possibility of losing the airway.

Instruments

1. Flexible. Fiberoptic bronchoscopes are available with an outer diameter of 3–6 mm. Light is transmitted through fiberoptic bundles, and the field of vision is usually 80°. They can be attached to a video camera for large screen display. The latest video bronchoscopes have a camera chip at the distal end of the scope.

2. Rigid. Rigid broncoscopes are available with a 3–9 mm diameter. Adult sizes are 7 mm in diameter and 40 cm in length. Telescopes with excellent optics are available for straight ahead (0°) viewing or at 30° and 90° for visualization of the upper lobe bronchi.

Pre-procedure evaluation

- History and physical examination.
- Bleeding time and prothrombin time (if coagulopathy is suspected).

Technique

1. Flexible bronchoscopy. A wide variety of techniques is used. The principles are listed below for an awake flexible bronchoscopy:

- NPO for 12 hours before procedure.
- Intravenous access.
- O_2 therapy, oxygen saturation monitoring.
- Sedation: e.g. Diazemuls 5–10 mg IV (optional).
- A drying agent such as atropine 0.3–0.6 mg (optional).
- Topical local anesthetic agents such as lidocaine (2%) applied to nasal, posterior pharyngeal mucosa and airway administered by spray, gargle or transcricoid injections. Additional lidocaine is administered directly through the bronchoscope as required (20 ml syringe containing 2–4 ml of 2% lidocaine and 16–18 ml air to flush).
- Nil by mouth (NPO) for 2–4 hours post-procedure until local anesthetic wears off to avoid aspiration.

The flexible bronchoscope may be introduced nasally or orally (using a mouth guard). Flexible bronchoscopy may also be performed through an endotracheal tube under general anesthesia. The proximal airway (larynx and trachea) is not generally visualized using this approach. Therefore, in collaboration with the anesthetist, the endotracheal cuff should be deflated, and the endotracheal tube withdrawn to the cords with the tip of the bronchoscope positioned just at the end of the tube.

2. *Rigid bronchoscopy*. Although rigid bronchoscopy can be carried out under local anesthesia, it is usually performed under general anesthesia in an operating room. After the rigid bronchoscope is introduced into the airway, a rigid lens system is used to visualize the airway in detail. Alternatively, a flexible bronchoscope can be passed through the rigid bronchoscope to visualize the segmental orifices. The limitations of rigid bronchoscopy include visualization of major lobar orifices only, and patient discomfort if performed under local anesthesia.

Potential complications of flexible bronchoscopy

- Respiratory depression, hypercarbia.
- Hypotension/syncope.
- Laryngospasm.
- Bronchospasm.
- Hypoxia.
- Arrhythmia.
- Aspiration.
- Allergic reaction to medication.
- Pneumothorax.
- Hemorrhage.
- Pneumonia.

Complications specific to rigid bronchoscopy

- Complications related to general anesthesia.
- Injury of the upper aerodigestive tract.
- Massive hemorrhage from large biopsy forceps.
- Subcutaneous emphysema or pneumonthorax from the use of high-pressure venturi ventilation.

Further reading

Cortese DA. Flexible bronchoscopy. In: Pearson FG, Deslauriers J, Ginsberg RJ, Hiebert CA, McKneally MF, Urschel HC, eds. *Thoracic Surgery*. New York: Churchill Livingstone, 1995; 200.

Feins RH, ed. Thoracic endoscopy. *Chest Surgery Clinics of North America*, 1996; **6**: 161.

Keshafjee S, Ginsberg RJ. Rigid bronchoscopy. In: Pearson FG, Deslauriers J, Ginsberg RJ, Hiebert CA, McKneally MF, Urschel HC, eds. *Thoracic Surgery*. New York: Churchill Livingstone, 1995; 190.

Related topics of interest

BULLOUS DISEASE AND EMPHYSEMA

Simon Pickard, Alan G. Casson

The indications and long-term results of surgical treatment for bullous disease and emphysema are evolving. Whereas bullectomy may benefit patients with an expanding solitary bulla, the value of surgery in generalized noncompressive disease is unclear. Lung transplantation has also been shown to benefit selected patients with emphysema. Although there has been considerable recent interest in lung volume reduction surgery, with encouraging early results suggesting improved functional and physiological parameters, the indications for surgery are unclear. To date, no randomized controlled trials have compared surgery with medical management.

Emphysema

Defined as an increase in the size of air spaces distal to the terminal nonrespiratory bronchiole, resulting in decreased expiratory flow rates, increased pulmonary resistance and over-inflation of the lung.

It is thought that these functional abnormalities result from inflammation of small conducting airways causing narrowing and premature closure. Destruction of lung tissue distal to the terminal bronchioles interferes with the supportive function of the peripheral airways, decreasing elastic recoil. The resulting hyperinflation of the lungs, with flattening of the diaphragm, impares the ability of the respiratory muscles to generate sufficient expiratory and inspiratory force. Dyspnoea increases as a result of awareness of increased neural stimulation to ventilate and eventual fatigue of respiratory muscles. The hyperinflated lungs act mechanically on both atria and ventricles, reducing diastolic filling, decreasing venous return and subsequently cardiac output.

1. Anatomic classification
- *Proximal acinar (centrilobular).* Respiratory bronchioles are enlarged and destroyed, typically due to smoking.
- *Panacinar (panlobular).* Involves uniform destruction of the entire acinus; associated with α_1-antitrypsin deficiency. Generally a more aggressive entity, with irregular involvement of the lungs.
- *Distal acinar (paraseptal).* Involves the distal part of the acinus and alveolus; associated with fibrosis, bullae and pneumothorax.

2. Clinical classification
- For the features of emphysema types A and B, see *Table 1*.
- *Compensatory emphysema.* Hyperinflation of a part of the lung secondary to lung loss. Strictly not true emphysema, as acinar destruction does not occur.
- *Bullous emphysema.* Associated with relatively normal underlying lung tissue; characterized by bulla or bleb formation.

Table 1. Features of emphysema types A and B

Parameter	Type A	Type B
Name	Emphysematous	Bronchitic
	Pink puffer	Blue bloater
Cough	Occasional	Severe
Sputum	Scant	Copious
Cyanosis	None	Frequent
Radiography	Bullae	Fibrosis
Airway resistance	Increased	Increased
Vital capacity	Normal/reduced	Reduced
Residual volume	Increased	Increased
Total lung capacity	Increased	Normal/reduced
PO_2	Normal/reduced	Reduced
PCO_2	Normal/reduced	Increased
Polycythemia	Rare	Frequent
Cor pulmonale	Rare	Frequent
Prognosis	Good	Poor
Pathology	Diffuse	Proximal acinar

- *Diffuse obstructive emphysema.* Synonymous with chronic obstructive lung disease.

Bullae

A bulla is an air-filled space within the lung parenchyma, resulting from intrinsic destruction of alveolar tissue. It has fibrous walls, and may communicate with the bronchial tree (open) or be isolated (closed). The degree to which bullae contribute to dyspnoea depends on the amount of lung tissue displaced and the extent of underlying disease.

Indications for surgery

- Moderate to severe dyspnoea.
- A localized bulla occupying >30% of the hemithorax.
- A progressively enlarging bulla.
- Complications of bullous disease (pneumothorax, infection, hemoptysis).

Preoperative assessment

1. Functional status. Clinical assessment is difficult because of a lack of objective methods to assess dyspnoea. Additionally, no single pulmonary function study will be adequate and therefore a panel of tests is usually performed, including gas transfer and total lung capacity. The forced expiratory volume in 1 s (FEV_1) appears to correlate with the size of the bulla, and therefore a disproportionately low value suggests diffuse disease. Arterial blood gases to document PaO_2 and $PaCO_2$.

2. Radiography. Old films are invaluable to assess the natural history and progression of bullae. Inspiratory and expiratory films may help differentiate localized bullous disease from emphysema.

3. CT scanning. This is the single most useful investigation to define the site, location and extent of bullae, and to assess the characteristics of the underlying lung and vasculature. It has generally replaced angiography and bronchography. Ventilation/perfusion lung scanning remains a useful investigation to quantitate functioning lung tissue.

Preoperative management

- Stop smoking.
- Chest physiotherapy.
- Consultation with respirologist.
- Antibiotics, bronchodilators and possibly steroids.
- Nutritional supplements.

Surgical procedures

1. Bullectomy. May be approached by median sternotomy, posterolateral thoracotomy or, more recently, by VATS. Pedunculated bullae are simply excised. Diffuse bullae are plicated, using the mechanical stapler, incorporating visceral pleura. Teflon or pericardium are often used to buttress the staple line to reduce air leakage. Potentially functional lung tissue should not be excised. Pleural synthesis (mechanical abrasion, pleurectomy) is an essential component of the procedure. Multiple chest tubes (connected to suction) may be required to maintain lung expansion postoperatively.

2. Pulmonary resection. Rarely required, but is the procedure of choice if a lobe is replaced by a large solitary bulla.

3. Laser ablation. Thoracoscopy with laser ablation, or electrocautery, was initially employed in high-risk patients with reported success. Largely surpassed by VATS and endo-stapling techniques.

4. Thoracostomy. Several variations of intracavity drainage (Monaldi procedures) have been described. These evolved as limited procedures to treat tuberculous cavities, and have subsequently been adapted for managing high-risk patients.

5. Lung volume reduction. Surgical resection of emphysematous lung appears to improve dyspnoea by reducing the work of breathing and improving gas exchange. Lung volume reduction surgery, comprising removal of 20–30% of lung volume, may achieve this by decreasing airway resistance, increasing lung elastic recoil, improving cardiac output and balancing ventilation/perfusion. The role of this approach is currently under intensive study.

6. Transplantation. Double lung transplantation has been utilized successfully in limited numbers of highly selected patients with end-stage lung disease. Long-term results are awaited.

Further reading

Deslauriers J, Leblanc P. Management of bullous disease. *Chest Surgery Clinics of North America*, 1994; **4:** 539.

Goldberg M. Emphysema and bullous disease. In: Pearson FG, Deslauriers J, Ginsberg RJ, Hiebert CA, McKneally MF, Urschel HC, eds. *Thoracic Surgery*. New York: Churchill Livingstone, 1995; 561.

Niederman MS, ed. Mechanisms and management of COPD. *Chest*, 1998; **113 (Suppl.):** 233S.

Related topics of interest

CARCINOID AND UNCOMMON LUNG TUMORS

Sean Grondin, Michael R. Johnston

Although NSCLC accounts for the vast majority of primary lung tumors, a few rare primary tumors may present with symptoms that mimic NSCLC, as a solitary pulmonary nodule or as an endobronchial lesion.

Carcinoid tumors

Account for approximately 5% of all lung cancers. Previously referred to as bronchial adenomas, implying (incorrectly) a benign prognosis. Pathologically, these tumors belong to the neuroendocrine group of tumors, known as the amine precursor uptake and decarboxylase (APUD) tumors, which arise from Kulchitzky cells of the respiratory epithelium. A spectrum of malignancy is seen. Typical carcinoids invade locally but have low malignant potential. Atypical carcinoids are characterized by increased mitotic activity and a tendency to metastasize. Small cell lung cancer is a highly malignant and rapidly fatal disease.

1. Typical carcinoid. This accounts for 90% of bronchial carcinoids. A well-differentiated neuroendocrine tumor, it consists of round or polygonal cells arranged in cords or clusters, with small nuclei and few mitoses, which rarely cause carcinoid syndrome. They invade locally, but have a low malignant potential (5–15% metastases). Carcinoids are highly vascular tumors that frequently bleed on bronchoscopic biopsy. However, this may be readily controlled by lavage with dilute epinephrine solution. These tumors are treated primarily by surgical resection. Segmental or wedge resections are indicated for small (<3 cm) peripheral lesions. For a central tumor, lobectomy (rarely pneumonectomy) or a bronchoplastic procedure should be considered, provided all disease is excised. Intraoperative frozen section is mandatory to examine resection margins (to within 5 mm of the tumor) and regional lymph nodes. Prognosis following a complete excision is excellent (>90% 10-year survival), and does not appear to be related to tumor size or the presence of lymph node metastases. Laser ablation of an endobronchial lesion is indicated only for palliation when the patient is a prohibitive operative risk for resection. Radiotherapy and chemotherapy are unhelpful with this disease.

2. Atypical carcinoid. A more aggressive variant characterized histologically by increased cellularity, pleomorphism, variable nuclear configuration and moderate mitotic activity. Metastases (predominantly regional lymph nodes) are reported in 50–70% of cases. Surgery is the treatment of choice for localized tumors, provided a complete resection is achieved. These tumors tend to be chemoresistant, with response rates generally below 30%.

Adenoid cystic carcinoma

Previously referred to as cylindroma, because of a characteristic tubular arrangement of cells. Generally slow growing, it infiltrates submucosa, perineural lymphatic channels and adjacent structures well beyond the visible extent of the tumor. This tumor is encountered most commonly in the trachea and major bronchi, where symptoms usually relate to airway obstruction. Diagnosis is made by bronchoscopic biopsy and bleeding is uncommon.

Complete surgical excision is the best treatment. The extent of resection depends on the location and extent of the tumor, and margins must be checked intraoperatively by frozen section. The presence of lymph node metastases does not preclude long-term survival if the resection is complete. Follow-up should be for 10–15 years at least. Palliation may be achieved by incomplete resection, debulking or preservation of the airway by laser or stenting. Radiotherapy may induce tumor regression and prevent local recurrence postoperatively. No effective chemotherapy regimen is known.

Mucoepidermoid carcinoma

Arises from minor salivary glands lining the tracheobronchial tree; may be confused with adenosquamous cancers histologically. Variable mitotic activity suggests different grades of malignancy: high-grade tumors typically metastasize to regional nodes, whereas low-grade tumors invade locally. This cancer is rare, arising most commonly in the trachea and major bronchi, producing symptoms of bronchial irritation or obstruction. Low-grade tumors should be excised completely, preserving as much normal lung tissue as possible (bronchoplastic procedures). High-grade tumors should be treated as NSCLC. Chemotherapy and radiotherapy are ineffective.

Pleomorphic mixed tumor

Rare; similar to salivary gland tumors. Epithelial cells are arranged in tubules or clusters, with variable stroma and occasional mitoses, the tumor tends to invade locally. Complete surgical excision is recommended.

Bronchial mucous gland adenoma

A truly benign tumor arising from mucous glands of the main bronchi. May be excised bronchoscopically or using bronchoplastic techniques.

Further reading

Burt M, Zakowski M. Rare primary malignant neoplasms. In: Pearson FG, Deslauriers J, Ginsberg RJ, Hiebert CA, McKneally MF, Urschel HC, eds. *Thoracic Surgery*. New York: Churchill Livingstone, 1995; 807.

Ducrocu X, Thomas P, Massard G, Barsotti P, Giudicelli R, Fuentes P, Wihlm JM. Operative risk and prognostic factors of typical bronchial carcinoid tumors. *Annals of Thoracic Surgery*, 1998; **65:** 1410.

Gould VE, Warren WH. The bronchopulmonary tract. In: Lechago J, Gould VE, eds. *Endocrine Pathology*. Baltimore: Williams and Wilkins, 1995.

Linnoila RI, Piantadosi S, Ruckdeschel JC. Impact of neuroendocrine differentiation in non-small cell lung cancer: the LCSG experience. *Chest*, 1994; **106:** 367S.

Warren WH, Memoli VA, Jordan AG. Reevaluation of pulmonary neoplasms resected as small cell carcinomas. Significance of distinguishing between well differentiated and small cell neuroendocrine carcinomas. *Cancer*, 1990; **65:** 1003.

Related topics of interest

CHEST TUBES

Chris Compeau, Michael R. Johnston

Chest tubes are generally inserted to evacuate collections of fluid, or air, from the pleural space, and to allow re-expansion of the underlying lung. Thoracic surgeons require a thorough understanding of chest-tube management, including the intricacies of the various drainage systems and potential complications related to their use.

Thoracic catheters

Available as straight or right-angled, thoracic catheters range in size from 6 F to 40 F and are made from silicone or plastic, with multiple drainage holes and a radiopaque line for radiographic localization. For most indications, at least a 28 F tube should be used. Smaller catheters (now often available in kits with a guidewire and dilator) are useful for neonates and for pneumothorax after needle lung biopsy.

Insertion technique

Several techniques are described, and should be selected according to patient need. The following key points should be considered for safe insertion of a chest tube under elective conditions. This technique has largely supplanted the use of external trocars. It is an invasive procedure and the patient therefore requires an explanation and must give informed consent. Premedicate with IM/IV narcotic at least 15–20 min prior to administering local anesthetic. Use a strict sterile technique, including a suitable skin antiseptic, and drape in a sterile manner. Locate the collection to be drained using a needle and syringe. For a loculated collection, localization by ultrasound is useful. This is an ideal time to take a sample of fluid for cytology, biochemistry or microbiology. The position of the tube is determined by the location and nature of the collection to be drained. However, the fifth or sixth intercostal space in the mid-axillary line is generally used for most situations, as minimal chest wall muscle is present. Inject local anesthetic at the proposed chest tube insertion site (skin, deeper tissues and parietal pleura), and wait to allow the anesthetic to work. This is not necessary for urgent insertion of a catheter in an unconscious patient. Ensure controlled spreading of intercostal muscles on the superior surface of rib, to avoid injury to the intercostal vessels and nerves. Entry into the (free) pleural space has a characteristic feel. This should be followed by digital exploration of the pleural cavity to assess pleural thickness, presence of nodules and adhesions. Insert the chest tube (at least 28 F), ensuring that the most proximal drainage hole is within the chest cavity, and connect to an underwater seal drainage system. Secure the chest tube to the chest wall with a nonabsorbable suture. Obtain a CXR to confirm the tube position.

Potential complications include pain, incorrect placement (extrapleural, in the fissure, drainage holes outside the pleura, tube kinked) and injury to intercostal vessels. Perforation of the lung, heart, aorta, vena cava, diaphragm, spleen, stomach and liver have all been reported, predominantly when trocar-directed tubes are used.

Drainage systems

Several drainage systems are available (commercially and in-house) and the thoracic surgeon should appreciate the advantages and limitations of each. The principle of closed drainage is, however, common to each. Normal intrapleural pressures (during spontaneous ventilation) range from $-8\,cmH_2O$ (inspiration) to $-2\,cmH_2O$ (expiration), but may be considerably lower or higher with forced inspiration or expiration, respectively.

1. Passive drainage system. This is an underwater seal drainage system of simple design. It employs positive expiratory pressure (the patient) and gravity to drain the pleural space. It may be connected to suction, but most central hospital systems are unreliable, and the pressures may vary widely. A disadvantage of the system is that as fluid accumulates in the bottle, the force required to overcome the underwater seal increases in proportion to the height of the water column. This may be a significant problem for an elderly patient with painful fractured ribs, for example, or for a patient with significant bleeding.

2. Active drainage systems. Based on the three-bottle system (*Figure 1*), comprising a collection chamber (which does not obstruct flow of fluid from the chest), an underwater seal (as above, which remains at a constant level, usually $2\,cmH_2O$) and a suction regulating device (to maintain constant negative

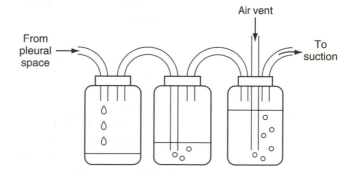

Figure 1. Three-bottle drainage system.

pressure, regardless of the source generating it). This system, applies continuous suction to the pleural space. with pressure settings generally ranging from -10 to $-20\,cmH_2O$. Various disposable units are available commercially, simple to use and are safe. A high-flow system (Emerson pump) may achieve a negative pressure of $-60\,cmH_2O$.

3. Portable valve systems. Several portable systems are available for selected patients with ongoing air leaks. These are based on a one-way flutter valve system, which theoretically may be advantageous as resistance to airflow is generally lower than with conventional underwater seal units. Occlusion of the flutter valve may occur if pleural fluid drainage persists and a collecting bag is usually required.

Chest tube management

1. Chest radiography. Essential to assess tube position, lung re-expansion, residual pleural fluid or pneumothorax.

2. Chest tube patency. Watch for respiratory fluctuations (approx. 6 cm) in the underwater seal fluid chamber. If there is no fluctuation, the tube is blocked. Consider removing the tube, repositioning the existing tube or inserting a new one. Excess fluid-filled loops of tubing should be avoided

3. Air leak. Bubbling in the underwater seal fluid chamber generally indicates an ongoing air leak, which may be continuous, present on one phase of spontaneous ventilation or only present on coughing. Check the system to exclude a leak in the chest tube/drainage system, by clamping the pleural drain just beyond its exit from the patient. If bubbling persists, there is a leak in the system. A vaseline-impregnated gauze can be placed around the tube at the skin exit site to prevent air from leaking into the chest through the tube tract.

4. Fluid drainage. Record the quantity and character of tube drainage per 24-hour period, or more frequently with hemothorax. Aim for a fluid output <150 ml/day prior to tube removal, although this is highly variable depending on the indication for chest drainage.

5. Chest tube removal. Remove the tube if it is not working, if there is no air leak and the lung is re-expanded. Fluid drainage should be minimal. Note that occasionally (i.e. following esophageal perforation, mediastinal surgery, etc.) chest tubes are left in place for prolonged periods. In this situation, the chest tube is not being used for its usual purpose, but rather to establish a drainage tract. Chest tube removal should take place on breath-holding, usually forced inspiration or expiration (depending on local custom). For ventilated patients, end-inspiration is preferred.

6. *Clamping chest tubes.* As a general rule, chest tubes should not be clamped. Exceptions to this rule are: when testing for system air leaks; when the drainage bottle requires replacement or has to be placed higher than the patient (to avoid fluid from the drainage bottle passing into the pleural space); and as a temporary measure to tamponade bleeding following a massive hemothorax, to avoid exsanguination while preparing for thoracotomy.

Further reading

Miller KS, Sahn SA. Chest tubes: indications, techniques, management and complications. *Chest*, 1987; **91:** 258.

Munnell ER. Thoracic drainage. *Annals of Thoracic Surgery*, 1997; **63:** 1497.

Ponn RB, Silverman HJ, Federico JA. Outpatient chest tube management. *Annals of Thoracic Surgery*, 1997; **64:** 1437.

Related topics of interest

CHEST-WALL RECONSTRUCTION

Chris Compeau, Michael R. Johnston

Chest-wall resection following trauma, infection or tumor may result in a large defect that requires reconstruction for physiologic reasons, to protect underlying thoracic viscera or for cosmesis. The location, size and depth of the defect are primary considerations. Reconstruction is frequently required after excision of four or more ribs, for full-thickness defects greater than 5 cm in diameter, particularly after resection of anterior or lateral lesions, and following sternectomy. Posterior or superior defects, deep to the body of the scapula (i.e. away from the tip), generally do not require reconstruction. Patients who receive preoperative radiotherapy should be evaluated carefully, as vascularity and wound healing may be compromised. Optimal results are often obtained with a multidisciplinary approach involving a plastic surgeon.

Bone reconstruction

Stabilization of the bony thorax may be achieved by the use of a synthetic prosthesis, provided the wound is not contaminated. Perioperative (prophylactic) antibiotics are administered routinely. Following implantation, fibrous tissue slowly infiltrates the interstices of the prosthetic material. Commonly available materials are:

- Polypropylene mesh. A double-stitch construction ensures rigidity in all directions.
- Polytetrafluoroethylene soft-tissue patch (2 mm). Impervious to fluid and air. Remains relatively expensive, however.
- Marlex mesh. Single-knit construction results in rigidity in one direction only, and therefore requires placement under tension in every direction.
- Marlex sandwich. Addition of methyl methacrylate (and steel mesh) between two layers of marlex, results in a rigid prosthesis.

Prostheses are sutured to the edges of the defect using monofilament nonabsorbable sutures in two layers. Soft tissues are closed over the prosthesis in layers to avoid a space where a seroma or hematoma may develop. Drains are not necessary and primary skin closure is preferred. Infection remains the major complication, which generally requires removal of the prosthesis. Reversible metabolic acidosis (due to anion release) has been reported when methacrylate is used.

Soft tissue reconstruction

1. Muscle. May be transposed alone, as a myocutaneous or as a free flap.

- *Latissimus dorsi.* Large flat muscle, with a well-defined neurovascular bundle (thoracodorsal), provides excellent coverage of chest-wall defects. May also be used as a musculocutaneous flap. Its secondary blood supply (artery to serratus anterior) may also be used as a basis for a flap.

- *Pectoralis major.* A good flap for anterior chest wall and sternal defects, based on its thoracoacromial neurovascular bundle, with minimal functional disability. Its secondary blood supply (perforating branches of the internal thoracic artery) may also be used as a basis for an alternative muscle flap.
- *Rectus abdominis.* Based on internal thoracic (superior epigastric), or inferior epigastric vessels, results in a versatile muscle or myocutaneous flap that may be orientated in several directions. It is particularly useful for lower sternal, anterior and inferior chest-wall defects.
- Other pedicle flaps may be based on serratus anterior (intrathoracic or combined with other muscle flaps), external oblique (lower thoracic defects) or trapezius (defects of the upper chest, base of neck, thoracic outlet).

2. *Omentum.* Based on the right or left gastroepiploic vessels; generally has an excellent blood supply. May be transposed over partial chest-wall defects, prostheses or into a previously irradiated or infected, area. It has no structural stability, and skin coverage (primary or graft) is essential.

Further reading

Seyfer AE, Graeber GM, eds. Chest wall reconstruction. *Surgery Clinics of North America*, 1989; **69:** 5.

Seyfer AE, Graeber GM, Wind G, eds. *Atlas of Chest Wall Reconstruction*. Rockville: Aspen, 1986.

Related topic of interest

Chest-wall tumors (p. 48)

CHEST-WALL TUMORS

Chris Compeau, Michael R. Johnston

Chest-wall tumors are rare. Approximately 50% are malignant, and of those, approximately half are primary tumors originating from tissues comprising the chest wall (i.e. bone, soft tissue, nerve, muscle). Although surgery still has a central role in diagnosis and management, multimodality therapy is used increasingly.

Evaluation

1. Clinical presentation. Often presents as an asymptomatic, slowly enlarging mass. Pain is present in 25–50% of cases and implies malignancy.

2. Tissue diagnosis. A definitive tissue diagnosis is essential. Previously, excisional biopsy was recommended as the 'gold standard'. Recent advances in histopathology (i.e. immunohistochemistry) now enable the pathologist to give a more accurate tumor diagnosis, particularly from smaller tissue samples.

- *Core needle biopsy.* Generally more accurate than fine-needle aspiration, but may not be diagnostic if the tumor is necrotic.
- *Incisional biopsy.* The incision should be planned for potential later excision at the time of a definitive tumor resection.
- *Excisional biopsy.* Performed if the lesion appears benign, or is small (i.e. <2–3 cm) and can be easily excised with normal tissue margins.

3. Staging. Radiographic imaging is used to determine the origin of the lesion, to evaluate potential metastases and to plan therapy. Plain CXR provide relatively limited information and CT scanning is the single most useful investigation. The role of magnetic resonance imaging (MRI) is currently under study. Occasionally, radionuclide bone scanning and angiography are required. Further evaluation of the cardiorespiratory system, coexisting disease, nutritional status, etc. may be required preoperatively.

Principles of treatment

The majority of primary malignant chest-wall tumors will require surgery. Wide excision is essential to obtain local control. This generally requires a margin of at least 4 cm of normal tissue on all sides ('without seeing the tumor'). Reconstruction of the chest wall may also be required, but should not compromise the extent of resection. For high-grade tumors of bone, the entire rib(s) should be excised, along with any attached structures (i.e. lung, pericardium, diaphragm, muscle, etc.). Increasingly, subsets of chest-wall tumors now receive pre- or postoperative chemotherapy or radiotherapy, although data from large, prospective clinical trials are lacking.

Benign primary chest-wall tumors

1. Chondroma. The most common benign chest-wall tumor. This arises anteriorly near the costochondral junction, and may grow to a large size and be occasionally painful. Chondroma is treated by local excision (with at least 2 cm margins).

2. Fibrous dysplasia. A painless mass arising in the posterior ribs of young adults, it has a radiologic appearance of an expanded mass with a thinned cortex and no calcification. Excisional biopsy is preferred for diagnosis. May be observed when typical radiologic appearance is present.

3. Osteochondroma. A rare tumor of young adults, it arises from the metaphysis, and grows in the opposite direction to the adjacent joint; covered with a cartilaginous cap. Solitary lesions are benign, while multiple lesions have malignant potential. The tumor is treated by wide local excision.

4. Eosinophilic granuloma. Arises from lymphoreticular tissue, and is not a true bone tumor. There is no malignant potential and excisional biopsy is preferred for diagnosis.

5. Desmoid tumor. Histologically similiar to a low-grade fibrosarcoma, it is usually well encapsulated. The tumor is slow growing and is associated with dull pain; there are no distant metastases. Desmoid tumors are treated by wide local excision (>4 cm margins) with chest-wall reconstruction. There are high rates of local recurrence although radiotherapy improves local control. Ten-year survival rates are >90%.

Malignant primary chest-wall tumors

1. Chondrosarcoma. The most common primary malignant chest-wall tumor, usually seen in adults. Eighty percent arise in the ribs (upper four), 20% in the sternum. Most are solitary lesions. Radiology shows a lobulated mass arising in the medulla, with cortical bone destruction and stippled calcification. The tumor is treated by wide local excision (>4 cm margins) with chest-wall reconstruction. Long-term prognosis depends on the tumor grade, size, location and extent of resection, 10-year survival is 96% with wide local excision, and 65% with local excision alone.

2. Ewing sarcoma. Neuroectodermal in origin, this tumor histologically comprises sheets of small, round, uniform, closely packed cells, with minimal cytoplasm; it is periodic acid–Schiff (PAS) positive. Askin's tumor is a highly malignant variant with characteristic chromosomal (11, 22) translocation. Ewing sarcoma occurs predominantly in children and adolescents and chest-wall pain (with or without a mass) is the predominant symptom. The patient may have leukocytosis and a raised sedimentation rate. There is a typical radiographic onion-peel appearance (due to multiple layers of periosteal new bone formation), bone destruction and a widened cortex and medulla. An incisional biopsy (with excision of the affected rib if possible) is essential. Combined modality treatment is now considered standard, with radiotherapy (local control) and chemotherapy (distant disease) using doxorubicin, dactinomycin, cyclophosphamide, and vincristine resulting in 5-year survival rates of >50%, with local control rates >90%.

3. *Osteosarcoma.* Presents as a painful rib mass in adolescents, or adults over 40 years. It may be associated with Paget's disease or previous chemoradiotherapy. A radiographic 'sunburst' pattern is seen, representing new periosteal bone formation. Triangular elevation of the periosteum (Codman's triangle) also occurs. An incisional biopsy is essential to establish a histologic diagnosis, and definitive therapy now comprises neoadjuvant chemotherapy (doxorubicin, methotrexate, cisplatin) followed by wide excision and reconstruction.

4. *Plasmacytoma.* Comprises 10–30% of all primary chest-wall malignancies and generally occurs in older males. Common sites for solitary lesions are the ribs, clavicle and sternum. The tumor presents radiographically as an osteolytic lesion, with soft tissue invasion, and further investigations include bone marrow aspiration and urine and skin immunoelectrophoreseis. A biopsy is required for diagnosis and definitive therapy of a solitary lesion is high-dose radiotherapy (50–60 Gy), with 5-year survival rates of 35–55%. Patients are at risk of developing multiple myeloma >10 years after diagnosis.

5. *Fibrosarcoma.* An uncommon soft-tissue sarcoma of the chest wall, it presents as a large painful chest-wall mass at any age, and radiography demonstrates an irregular soft-tissue lesion with bone destruction. Metastases to the lung are common. Low-grade tumors are treated by wide local excision and reconstruction, whereas high-grade sarcomas require wide local excision with adjuvant chemotherapy. Five-year survivals range from 50 to 80%.

6. *Rhabdomyosarcoma.* A rare tumor of mesodermal origin. Immunohistochemistry is useful to detect tumor markers (myoglobin, desmin, myosin, actin). The tumor is treated by wide local excision and multidrug chemotherapy.

7. *Malignant fibrous histiocytoma (MFH).* A rare tumor arising from histiocytes. It shows frequent local recurrence and metastasis, and is treated by wide local excision and radiotherapy.

8. *Liposarcoma.* Usually a low-grade tumor, this is treated by wide local excision and has a 5-year survival of >80%.

Metastatic chest-wall tumors

A solitary metastasis to the chest wall may occur from primary thyroid, colonic, genitourinary and sarcomatous malignancies. Renal cell and thyroid malignancies may metastasize to the sternum, and present as a pulsatile mass. Resection of a single metastasis should be considered.

Further reading

Burt M. Primary malignant tumors: the Memorial Sloan-Kettering Cancer Center experience. *Chest Surgery Clinics of North America*, 1994; **4:** 137.

Pass HI. Primary and metastatic chest wall tumors. In: Roth JA, Ruckdeschel JC, Weisenburger TH, eds. *Thoracic Oncology*, 2nd edn. Philadelphia: WB Saunders, 1995; 519.

Related topic of interest

Chest-wall reconstruction (p. 46)

CHYLOTHORAX

Chris Compeau, Michael R. Johnston

Chylothorax is the abnormal accumulation of lymphatic fluid in the pleural space. This usually occurs as a result of a leak from the thoracic duct or one of its major tributaries.

Anatomy of the thoracic duct

The duct orginates intra-abdominally from the cisterna chyli, located prevertebrally at the level of L1 or L2. It then passes superiorly through the aortic hiatus and extrapleurally along the right anterior surface of the vertebral bodies, medial to the azygous vein and posterior to the esophagus (azygo-esophageal recess). At the T5 to T7 vertebral level the duct crosses to the left side, posterior to the esophagus. It then proceeds cephalad behind the aortic arch and left subclavian artery. Above the clavicle, the duct turns laterally behind the carotid sheath, anterior to the inferior thyroid, vertebral and subclavian arteries. At the medial margin of scalenus anterior it turns inferiorly to enter the venous system at the left subclavian–internal jugular vein junction. Thoracic duct anatomy is said to be 'consistent in its inconsistency', with the 'classic' anatomy (above) found in only 50% of patients.

Composition of thoracic duct lymph (chyle)

Lymphatic vessels collect and transport tissue fluids, extravasated plasma proteins, absorbed lipids (chylomycrons) and other large macromolecules from the intestine to the intravascular space. In addition, lymphocytes also circulate through this system.

- Milky white (clear when fasting), odorless, sterile on culture.
- Alkaline pH 7.4–7.8.
- Rate of lymph flow varies with fat consumption (0.38–3.9 ml/min).
- Total fat = 14–210 mM.
- Triglycerides, chyle > plasma (medium chain triglycerides absorbed directly from the small intestines into the portal venous system).
- Cholesterol, chyle < plasma.
- Cholesterol/triglyceride ratio <1.
- Total protein = 21–59 g/l; albumin = 12–42 g/l.
- Lymphocytes = 400–6800 $\times$ 10^6/l – the principal cellular element.
- Erthrocytes = 50–600 $\times$ 10^6/l (similiar to plasma composition).
- Electrolytes = plasma.

Etiology

1. *Congenital.* Rare, usually presents in the neonatal period, and is related to birth trauma and/or developmental duct abnormalities.

2. *Traumatic.* Mechanism of injury following blunt trauma is spinal hyperextension resulting in direct rupture of the duct above diaphragm. Penetrating injuries are rare. Injuries above T5 generally result in a left chylothorax, whereas injuries below T5 generally result in a right chylothorax.

3. *Operative.* A relatively common mechanism of injury, complicating any thoracic or cardiovascular surgical procedure. The duct is most susceptible to injury in upper left chest (i.e. during surgery of the aortic arch, subclavian artery or esophagus), and at the aortic hiatus (i.e. during transhiatal esophagectomy, aortic aneurysm repair).

4. *Neoplastic.* Intrinsic or extrinsic thoracic duct obstruction, secondary to thoracic malignancy (most commonly lymphomas), may cause distension and rupture of the thoracic duct, resulting in a 'spontaneous' chylothorax. Direct invasion may occasionally occur, particularly with the epithelial tumors (i.e. lung or esophageal cancer). Chylothorax may rarely be associated with benign tumors (i.e. lymphangioma, mediastinal hygroma).

5. *Infectious.* Rarely, tuberculous lymphadenitis, filiarisis or ascending lymphangitis, may result in chylothorax. The pathophysiology is generally thought to be related to duct obstruction.

6. *Miscellaneous*
   - Spontaneous. Violent coughing or vomiting, resulting in a shearing effect at the right diaphragmatic crus.
   - Venous thrombosis. Superior vena cava (SVC), left subclavian or jugular veins.
   - Pulmonary lymphangiomyomatosis.
   - Idiopathic.

Clinical presentation

1. *Postoperative.* A milky chest tube drainage at 24–72 hours (occasionally longer), usually on resumption of oral intake.

2. *Nonoperative.* Progressive shortness of breath with physical and radiological evidence of a pleural effusion. Following chest tube drainage (or repeated thoracentesis), fluid losses may be significant (>2500 ml/day), resulting in cardiovascular instability. Protein, fat-soluble vitamin and antibody losses may have nutritional and immunologic consequences.

Diagnosis

A high index of suspicion should be maintained. Long-standing pleural effusions may have a chylous appearance, as may cholesterol effusions associated with tuberculosis or rheumatoid arthritis. These do not contain chylomycrons or fat globules.

1. Thoracentesis

2. Pleural fluid analysis
- Gram stain, lymphocytosis (>90%); no bacteria.
- Sudan III stain, fat globules; microscopy, free fat; fat content > plasma.
- Lipid analysis, cholesterol/triglyceride ratio <1.
- Triglyceride level >1.24 mM.
- Lipoprotein electrophoresis, chylomicrons.

3. Radionuclide scanning. Scanning with ^{99}Tc antimony sulfide colloid may demonstrate the level of thoracic duct obstruction and site of leakage.

4. Lymphangiography. This may also demonstrate the site of obstruction and leakage. This study may be performed to define thoracic-duct anatomy if surgery is planned.

5. CT scanning. Used to define associated thoracic pathology (i.e. mediastinal tumor).

Management

The aims of treatment are to drain the pleural space, ensure expansion of the underlying lung and to reduce the volume of thoracic-duct leakage. The timing of operative intervention remains somewhat controversial and depends on the cause of the chylothorax and the daily volume of drainage. There are no known adverse sequelae to ligation of the intrathoracic portion of the thoracic duct. In addition, consideration should be given to treatment of the underlying cause (i.e. tumor, or preventing the development of a chylothorax at the initial procedure).

1. Conservative. Conservative management involves: (i) chest tube drainage (preferred to repeated thoracentesis) of the pleural space; (ii) NPO, (enteral formulae with low fat content and medium chain triglycerides are recommended but rarely work in practice); and (iii) total parenteral nutrition, with correction of fluid and electrolyte imbalance.

2. Operative. Previous estimates suggested that 50% of leaks would close spontaneously with 14 days of conservative management. However, a shorter period of nonsurgical management is recommended to avoid the fluid and nutritional consequences of ongoing leakage. Consistent daily drainage of 1000 ml (adults) or 100 ml/year of age (children) over 5–7 days would suggest early surgical intervention. Several operative approaches are reported. Operative identification of the thoracic duct may be facilitated by instilling 100–300 ml of cream or olive oil into the stomach (via a nasogastric tube), 1 hour preoperatively.

For patients in whom the risk of surgery is acceptable, right thoracotomy and mass ligation of the thoracic duct above the right hemidiaphragm is the preferred approach, and is successful in over 80% of patients. Nonabsorbable sutures (with pledgets) are used to ligate all tissues in the azygo-esophageal recess. Occasionally large metal clips may be useful, particularly with thoracoscopic approaches. Although an extrapleural approach is described, it offers few advantages over a transpleural approach. A parietal pleurectomy is generally performed at the time of thoracotomy, to ensure pleural synthesis (and therefore tamponade any additional pleural drainage not controlled by the mass ligation). Chest-tube drainage (with suction) is maintained for several days postoperatively.

Thoracoscopic approaches are used increasingly, but require further evaluation. Direct ligation (open or thoracoscopic) of the leaking duct is generally not effective. A pleuroperitoneal shunt may be useful for control of diffuse leakage, or when multiple thoracic duct channels preclude effective mass ligature above the diaphragm. Miscellaneous procedures (i.e. anastomosis of the thoracic duct to the azygous vein, fibrin glue, radiotherapy, pleurodesis with talc) are reported with variable success.

Further reading

Johnstone DW, Feins RH. Chylothorax. *Chest Surgery Clinics of North America*, 1994; **4:** 617.
Malthaner RA, McKneally MF. Anatomy of the thoracic duct and chylothorax. In: Pearson FG, Deslauriers J, Ginsberg RJ, Hiebert CA, McKneally MF, Urschel HC, eds. *Thoracic Surgery*. New York: Churchill Livingstone, 1995; 1069.
Miller JI. Diagnosis and management of chylothorax. *Chest Surgery Clinics of North America*, 1996; **6:** 139.

Related topics of interest

Chest tubes (p. 42)
Pleural effusion (p. 197)

CONGENITAL BRONCHOPULMONARY ANOMALIES

Simon Pickard, Alan G. Casson

Congenital bronchopulmonary malformations are rare. They may present in various ways as life-threatening lesions at birth, as incidental radiographic findings in children and adults, or as a lung mass in patients with recurrent pulmonary infections or bronchiectasis.

Embryology

The median pharyngeal groove, from which the paired lung buds arise, appears on the primitive foregut (endoderm) at 22 days. The lung buds grow caudally into the mesochyme independent of the esophagus, and the mesenchymal septum separating these structures persists throughout development. By the eighth week, a distinct lobar architecture is recognized, with a defined vasculature. From the 8 th to 16 th week, the bronchial divisions are established and proliferate rapidly. From 4 to 6 months, respiratory bronchioles and alveoli develop, with mature alveolar cells (type 1 and 2 pneumocytes). After birth, there is a ninefold increase in the number of terminal alveoli (predominantly during the first year) up to 12 years of age.

It should be appreciated that often no correlation exists between patterns of congenital anomalies and the sequence of embryologic development, suggesting a multifactorial etiology for many of the following malformations.

Tracheal atresia/agenesis

This condition is rare. Neonates may be premature, with a history of polyhydramnios. They present with respiratory distress at birth. Attempts at intubation are unsuccessful, although mask ventilation often results in improved oxygenation (via esophago-bronchial communication). There is no suitable surgical treatment for tracheal agenesis and multiple congenital anomalies are often present. In neonates with tracheal atresia, immediate tracheostomy is used if the distal airway is normal, and repair may be possible.

Bronchial anomalies

Anomalies of tracheo-bronchial budding occur at day 26, and are thought to result in bronchial atresia, congenital bronchiectasis and lobar emphysema. Esophageal atresia and tracheoesophageal fistulae are often associated.

1. Bronchial atresia. Results in obstruction to the flow of pulmonary secretions, which form a mucocele proximal to the atresia. May remain asymptomatic. Recurrent pulmonary infection is an indication for resection.

2. Congenital bronchiectasis. Bronchi distal to the second or third divisions have insufficient cartilage and remain cystic, resulting in recurrent pneumonia. Localized disease may be resected successfully.

3. Congenital lobar emphysema. Idiopathic hyperinflation of one lobe (usually left upper), causing severe respiratory distress in infancy. Chest X-ray demonstrates overinflation of a lobe, with mediastinal shift. No specific bronchial obstruction is demonstrated. It is speculated that the cause of air-trapping and hyperinflation is related to intrinsic weakness of the supporting cartilage, possibly in association with some degree of extrinsic compression by related vascular structures. Urgent lobectomy is curative.

4. Anomalous bronchi. May rarely connect to the foregut, proximal airway (tracheal bronchus) or biliary tree.

Sequestration

Segments of nonfunctional lung that have no bronchial communication with the airway or other foregut derivative. Arterial blood supply is systemic, usually directly from the aorta. Venous return is to the pulmonary veins in the majority of cases. Should be differentiated from accessory pulmonary lobes, which maintain normal communication to the tracheobronchial tree.

1. Extralobar. Usually asymptomatic, as air spaces are not present. Presents as an incidental finding, characteristically as a triangular shadow in the posterior costophrenic angle adjacent to the aorta or esophagus. Excision is usually required for diagnosis. Care should be taken to define the blood supply to the lesion.

2. Intralobar. Most common in the lower lobes (left > right) and may contain air spaces. Presents with recurrent pneumonia and abscess formation. Vascular sequaelae may result from high systemic blood flow into the pulmonary system (i.e. hemoptysis, congestive heart failure, enlarging mass on serial CXR). Often requires lobectomy.

Pulmonary aplasia/agenesis

Complete absence of pulmonary parenchyma and vasculature on the affected side. The only difference between aplasia and agenesis is the presence of a rudimentary bronchus to the aplastic lung. Associated congenital heart disease is common, especially for right-sided lesions. Most infants who survive 5 years (50%) can expect a normal life span.

Pulmonary hypoplasia

1. Primary. Very rare. Thought to result from fetal pulmonary hypertension, resulting in increased pulmonary arterial smooth muscle, and an exaggerated vasoconstrictive response to hypoxia and acidosis. Neonates present with respiratory distress and the CXR reveals small, clear lungs. Despite treatment of pulmonary vasoconstriction and hypertension, mortality rates are high.

2. *Secondary.* Associated with a wide spectrum of maternal and fetal abnormalities.

- *Oligohydramnios.* Renal agenesis, dysplasia.
- *Bone dysplasias* (*small, rigid chest*). Achondroplasia, osteogenesis imperfecta, neonatal hypophosphatemia.
- *Decreased fetal respiratory movements.* Arthrogryposis multiplex, myotonic dystrophy.
- *Diaphragmatic elevation.* Eventration, ascites, abdominal tumor, phrenic nerve agenesis.
- *Thoracic lesions.* Congenital diaphragmatic hernia, congenital cystic adenomatoid malformation (CCAM), mediastinal tumors, enteric duplication cysts.
- *Pulmonary vascular anomalies.* Pulmonary artery agenesis, Scimitar syndrome.
- *Miscellaneous.* Omphalocele, Down's syndrome.

Pulmonary parenchymal disease

1. *Bronchogenic cysts.* Cyst walls are lined by ciliated columnar or cuboidal epithelium, and may contain cartilage and mucous glands. They often communicate with the bronchial lumen, and may be single, multiple or multiloculated, they are located in the pulmonary parenchyma (esp. lower lobes), mediastinum or hilum. Pulmonary cysts present with recurrent infection, mediastinal cysts with airway obstruction. Hemoptysis occurs infrequently and definitive treatment is by excision.

2. *Congenital cystic adenomatoid malformation (CCAM).* Characterized by disorganized overgrowth of terminal bronchiolar-type structures, with lack of mature alveoli. Lesions may be solid or cystic and are localized to one lobe, rarely an entire lung. CCAM presents clinically as: (i) stillborn infants (solid lesion); (ii) premature neonate with respiratory distress (mixed cystic/solid lesion); (iii) older infant/child with recurrent pulmonary infection or pneumothorax (cystic lesion). The lesion shows variable radiographic patterns (solid/cystic), and should be distinguished from congenital lobar emphysema or diaphragmatic hernia. Surgical resection (i.e. lobectomy or segmentectomy) is curative.

3. *Hamartomas/tumors.* A benign tumor-like malformation which contains disordered but mature pulmonary tissues. Congenital tumors are otherwise rare.

Pulmonary vascular anomalies

1. *Scimitar syndrome.* The right pulmonary veins drain into the inferior vena cava (IVC) or right atrium, leading to a characteristic radiographic appearance. Associated with a range of anomalies, including hypoplasia of the right lung, dextroposition of the heart, congenital heart disease, hypoplasia of the

right pulmonary artery, an anomalous systemic blood supply to the lung, congenital diaphragmatic hernia, hemivertebrae and imperforate anus. Children may be asymptomatic, or present with congestive heart failure secondary to the left-to-right shunt or recurrent respiratory infection. Embolization of anomalous arteries, operative ligation of venous return and right pneumonectomy are reported.

2. *Arteriovenous fistulae.* May be solitary or multiple. Sixty percent occur in the lower lobes, unilaterally. Forty percent are associated with the Osler–Weber–Rendu syndrome. Recurrent pulmonary infection, cyanosis, dyspnoea and hemoptysis may occur at any age. The vascular anatomy is defined by angiography. Now with concurrent embolization. Surgical resection is rarely necessary.

3. *Lymphangiectasia.* May be generalized or limited to the lungs. Primary pulmonary disease is associated with Noonan's syndrome. Secondary lymphangiectasis results from obstruction to pulmonary venous outflow, with total anomalous venous return, aortic/mitral atresia. Treatment is supportive.

4. *Pulmonary artery agenesis.* Pulmonary hypoplasia is present on the affected side, with systemic arterial blood supply and a normal pulmonary venous return. May present in adults with hemoptysis and bronchiectasis, for which resection should be performed. Pulmonary artery agenesis may also be associated with Swyer–James syndrome (unilateral pulmonary hyperlucency without lobar inflation).

Further reading

Azizkhan RG. Congenital pulmonary lesions in childhood. *Chest Surgery Clinics of North America*, 1993; **3:** 547.

Luck SR, Reynolds M, Raffensperger JG. Congenital bronchopulmonary malformations. In: Ravitch MM, Steichen FM, eds. *Current Problems in Surgery*. Chicago: Year Book Medical Publishers, 1986; 251.

Pegolio W, Mattei P, Colombani PM. Congenital intrathoracic vascular abnormalities in childhood. *Chest Surgery Clinics of North America*, 1993; **3:** 529.

Related topics of interest

CORROSIVE ESOPHAGEAL INJURY

Donna E. Maziak, F. Griff Pearson

Corrosive injury to the esophagus may result from accidental (usually children) or deliberate (usually adolescents or adults) ingestion of strong acid or alkali. The resulting injury (coagulation necrosis from acid, liquefaction necrosis from alkali) to the esophageal mucosa may result in superficial or deep burns, stricture or perforation. Whereas accidental ingestion of a small volume of corrosive may result only in oropharyngeal injury, deliberate ingestion of a large volume may result in injury at any level of the foregut. Accurate diagnosis and early evaluation of the extent of injury are essential for successful management.

Initial management

1. *Diagnosis.* The exact nature of the ingested substance should be determined. A thorough history and physical examination are performed, with particular attention to exclude injury to the airway or esophageal perforation. All patients suspected of ingesting caustic materials should be admitted to hospital for further assessment. Intravenous fluids and antibiotics are administered as necessary.

2. *Endoscopy.* The timing of endoscopy was previously controversial. However, most surgeons now favor early examination, under general anesthesia. Initially the oropharynx is evaluated directly and suspicion of airway injury mandates bronchoscopy. The foregut is examined carefully using a pediatric flexible fiberoptic gastroscope. Injury is minimized by only advancing the instrument to the first level of burn, with minimal air insufflation.

3. *Oropharyngeal injury.* If only the oropharynx is involved, IV fluids are given until oral intake is resumed. Severe injury, particularly in children, may result in stricture formation, particularly around the mouth. Although oral stents have been proposed to reduce the degree of stricturing, plastic surgery may be required.

4. *Laryngotracheal injury.* This should be determined early to avoid airway compromise. Patients exhibiting respiratory obstruction resulting from airway edema should undergo tracheotomy. Subsequent stricture may be managed by dilation, although a few patients may require a permanent tracheostome.

5. *Esophageal injury.* This generally occurs with associated mouth burns. Endoscopic assessment of the depth of injury may predict healing. Administration of steroids has not been shown to prevent the development of stricture.
   Superficial burns are characterized by erythema and edema of the mucosa, with ulceration less than the circumference of

the esophagus. Intravenous fluids and antibiotics are given until patients are able to handle their secretions and swallow without pain. Liquids (nonacidic) are started and a soft diet advanced as tolerated. The endoscopy is repeated at 2–3 weeks to evaluate healing and to examine the entire foregut. Any early strictures are dilated carefully at this time. A barium swallow may be performed at this stage.

Full-thickness burn injuries are characterized by sloughing of the mucosa, often with associated circumferential ulceration. If the injury appears severe, a mini-laparotomy should be considered to place a feeding jejunostomy. A gastrostomy (high on the lesser curve to avoid compromising use of the stomach if esophageal replacement becomes necessary) is an alternative, especially if retrograde dilation is to be performed later. Otherwise IV antibiotics and fluids are administered until the patient stops drooling and is able to swallow saliva pain-free. Repeated clinical (and radiologic) observation is essential during this time, to exclude perforation. As stricturing is likely following full-thickness injury, the esophagus is reassessed by barium swallow and endoscopy 3 weeks after the initial injury. Dilation is initiated at this stage and the patient started on liquids, progressing to a soft diet as tolerated. The frequency of dilation varies, but generally averages every 2 weeks. This may eventually be performed under local anesthesia as an outpatient procedure, or by the patient at home. If at 6 months there is no response to dilation, the esophagus may need to be replaced. The role of esophageal stenting is unclear.

6. *Perforation.* Esophageal or gastric perforation with associated mediastinitis or peritonitis is relatively uncommon, but should be treated aggressively. As repair of the damaged esophagus or stomach is rarely possible, resection is frequently life-saving. Reconstruction of the foregut is generally performed electively several months later.

Follow-up and late management

Long-term follow-up is essential to detect and manage the following complications of corrosive esophageal injury.

- Restricturing.
- Gastroesophageal reflux and associated complications (esophagitis, peptic stricture, aspiration, etc.).
- Chronic aspiration pneumonias and bronchiectasis.
- Nutritional deficiency.
- Malignancy.

Failure of medical therapy and dilation to manage these complications, to improve swallowing and quality of life, suggests surgery to resect and replace the esophagus may be the only satisfactory option.

1. Preoperative. Careful attention is given to nutritional status and hydration. Previous airway injuries are re-evaluated, with particular attention to vocal-cord function and to exclude subglottic stenosis. The extent of foregut injury is also re-evaluated by barium swallow and endoscopy. Esophageal function studies (i.e. manometry and ambulatory 24-hour pH) may be used to document the degree of esophageal dysfunction.

2. Resection. Dense mediastinal fibrosis is generally present and a transthoracic approach (not transhiatal) is warranted. The esophageal mobilization may be technically challenging and sharp dissection is a useful technique. If the dissection is felt to be too hazardous, esophageal bypass should be considered.

3. Reconstruction. Stomach is the preferred substitute, assuming no previous injury. Isoperistaltic colon interposition is also a durable long-term substitute, but is a technically demanding operation. The posterior mediastinal (orthotopic) route is the most direct, but a substernal route is also satisfactory, provided the thoracic inlet is enlarged by resecting the medial clavicle and first rib.

Further reading

Andreoni B, Farina ML, Biffi R, Crosta C. Emergency management of caustic ingestion. *Diseases of the Esophagus*, 1997; **10**: 95.

Estrara A, Taylor W, Mills LJ, Platt MR. Corrosive burns of the esophagus and stomach: a recommendation for an aggressive surgical approach. *Annals of Thoracic Surgery*, 1986; **41**: 276.

Kirsh MM, Ritter F. Caustic ingestion and subsequent damage to the oropharyngeal and digestive passages. *Annals of Thoracic Surgery*, 1976; **21**: 74.

Zagar SA, Kochhar R, Hehta S, Mehta SK. The role of fibreoptic endoscopy in the management of corrosive ingestion and modified endoscopic classification of burns. *Gastrointestinal Endoscopy*, 1991; **37**: 165.

Related topics of interest

CRICOPHARYNGEAL DISORDERS

Donna E. Maziak, F. Griff Pearson

Oropharyngeal dysphagia represents a symptom complex, comprising difficulty in swallowing localized to the neck, often associated with oral or nasal regurgitation, aspiration and voice change. Although it is a relatively common symptom of patients presenting to the ear, nose and throat (ENT) or thoracic surgical clinic, it is difficult to evaluate objectively. The etiology of oropharyngeal dysphagia is quite extensive, but generally arises as a consequence of neurologic or neuromuscular disorders of the upper esophageal sphincter. However, gastroesophageal reflux disease and other esophageal motility disorders may also result in symptoms referred to the neck.

Etiology and classification

1. *Neurogenic*
   - *Central.* Vascular event, multiple sclerosis, amyotrophic lateral sclerosis, bulbar disease, Parkinson's disease, tumors, trauma.
   - *Peripheral.* Neuropathy from alcohol or diabetes, tumor, trauma.

2. *Myogenic.* Muscular or endplate disease.

3. *Upper esophageal sphincter dysfunction*
   - Idiopathic, isolated cricopharyngeal dysfunction.
   - Associated pharyngoesophageal diverticulum (Zenker's diverticulum).

4. *Iatrogenic.* Following surgery or radiotherapy.

5. *Distal esophageal dysfunction.* Referred from gastroesophageal reflux disease, various motor disorders, or mechanical obstruction (i.e. stricture).

6. *Mechanical.* Local neck pathology causing intrinsic or extrinsic compression.

7. *Psychogenic*

Investigations

1. *History and physical examination.* The nature and severity of symptoms do not necessarily correlate with objective findings and considerable clinical judgement may be necessary to assess patients presenting with cricopharyngeal dysphagia.

2. *Video esophagogram.* To delinate any anatomic or functional abnormalities of the oropharynx and upper esophagus during the early phase of swallowing.

3. *Endoscopic examination.* Initially, panendoscopy of the oropharynx, larynx and upper esophagus using rigid instrumentation, followed by flexible fiberoptic esophagogastroscopy to evaluate anatomic abnormalities and coexisting mucosal disease (i.e. tumor, esophagitis) of the foregut.

4. Esophageal function studies. Manometric evaluation of the upper esophageal sphincter is technically difficult because of radial asymmetry and the degree of movement during swallowing. Recent advances with multiple port catheters or solid-state sensors may provide a more accurate diagnosis in the future. Evaluation of the esophageal body and lower esophageal sphincter is performed to exclude associated esophageal motor disorders. Ambulatory 24-hour pH monitoring is carried out to evaluate acid reflux.

5. Radionuclide transit studies. Provide semi-quantitative information about solid and liquid transit. However, further validation of this investigation and standardization between centers, is warranted. This investigation is not used routinely.

Management

It is essential that as precise a diagnosis as possible is established before treatment is initiated. Local causes (i.e. tumors) and associated disorders (i.e. gastroesophageal reflux disease) should be treated separately. In general, medical management and dilation have little role in the management of neurologic or myogenic disorders. Carefully selected patients may benefit from surgery (i.e. myotomy) to reduce resistance to swallowing, especially if hypertension, incomplete relaxation or dysfunction of the upper esophageal sphincter, is documented objectively.

1. Upper esophageal myotomy. This may be performed under local or general anesthesia. A left neck approach is preferred to the cervical esophagus. The cricoid cartilage is used to locate the pharyngo-esophageal junction. Finger retraction (left lobe of thyroid) minimizes injury to the left recurrent laryngeal nerve (in the tracheo-esophageal groove). The myotomy extends across cricopharyngeus (occasionally a very prominent muscle) for a variable distance (usually 4–6 cm; but controversial) onto the upper esophageal body. A bougie is helpful to stent the esophagus during the procedure. A strip of muscle is usually sent for histopathology. A nasogastric tube and neck drains are not generally required. Patients have a water-soluble (followed by dilute barium) contrast study the following day (to exclude a mucosal leak), and are started on liquids and progressed to solids over 2–3 days, prior to discharge from hospital. Complications specific to this procedure are recurrent laryngeal nerve trauma; esophageal mucosal injury, with consequent neck or mediastinal infection; and salivary fistula, retropharyngeal hematoma, and aspiration. Results, in carefully selected patients, are generally reported to be good to excellent in terms of quality of swallowing. However, relatively small patient numbers, various etiologic factors and nonstandardized methods of evaluating swallowing make evaluation of results difficult. Intact voluntary swallowing, adequate mobility of the tongue, normal phonation and the absence of dysarthria appear to be predictive of a good surgical outcome.

Further reading

Duranceau A. Pharyngeal and cricopharyngeal disorders. In: Pearson FG, Deslauriers J, Ginsberg RJ, Hiebert CA, McKneally MF, Urschel HC, eds. *Esophageal Surgery*. New York: Churchill Livingstone, 1995; 389.

Ekberg O, Olsson R. The pharyngoesophageal segment: functional disorders. *Diseases of the Esophagus*, 1995; **8**: 252.

Lerut T, Coosemans W, Cuypers P, DeLeyn P, Deneffe G, Migliore M, Van Raemdonck D. The pharyngoesophageal segment: cervical myotomy as theraupetic principle for pharyngoesophageal disorders. *Diseases of the Esophagus*, 1996; **9**: 22.

Orringer MB. Extended cervical esophagomyotomy for cricopharyngeal dysfunction. *Journal of Thoracic and Cardiovascular Surgery*, 1980; **80**: 669.

Related topics of interest

DIAPHRAGM

Gail Darling

The diaphragm is a musculoaponeurotic structure separating the thoracic and abdominal cavities, and is a major muscle of respiration. Contraction of the diaphragm results in a shortening and flattening of the central tendon, increasing the volume of the thoracic cavity and reducing intrapleural pressure (inspiration). Relaxation results in restoration of its characteristic domed configuration, with consequent reduction of intrathoracic volume (expiration). These involuntary cyclical changes are essential for spontaneous ventilation.

Surgical anatomy

The peripheral muscular portion originates from the following, which insert into a central aponeurosis (tendon).

- Sternum, comprising two muscular slips arising from the xiphoid, inserting anteriorly.
- Costal muscle bundles, from the lower six costal cartilages, interdigitating with transversus abdominis, inserting anterolaterally.
- Medial and lateral arcuate ligaments, thickened fascia overlying the psoas and quadratus lumborum muscles, inserting posteriorly.
- Crura, posterior muscle bundles arising from the bodies and intervertebral disks of L1–L3 (right) and L1–L2 (left). The medial fibres decussate to form the median arcuate ligament overlying the aortic hiatus (T12), which also transmits the thoracic duct and azygous veins. The right crus encircles the esophagus and vagi (T10) and inserts posteriorly into the central tendon.

The phrenic nerves (C3,4,5) provide sensory and motor function, and penetrate the diaphragm just lateral to the caval foramina (T8) (right phrenic nerve) and lateral to the left heart border (left phrenic nerve). Both nerves branch on the inferior surface of the diaphragm below the peritoneal surface. The arterial supply of the diaphragm arises from paired phrenic arteries (arising from the abdominal aorta), musculophrenic and pericardiophrenic arteries (internal thoracic arteries) and the intercostals. Venous drainage is analogous to the arterial supply, but is more variable.

Incisions are required for various abdominal or thoracic procedures, and should be made with care to avoid damage to branches of the phrenic nerve and associated vascular structures.

A circumferential incision is made approximately 2 cm parallel to the chest wall (no less, as closure may prove difficult). This is a safe incision, which provides excellent exposure in most situations, with minimal impairment of respiratory function. It is useful to place marking sutures to ensure correct orientation of the diaphragm during closure. Radial, midline and paracardiac (or medial) incisions are described, but should not extend too far medially to avoid transecting major branches of the phrenic nerve.

Multiple, interrupted, heavy (0 or No.1), nonabsorbable sutures, in a figure-of-eight or mattress pattern, were classically recommended to close diaphragmatic incisions. However, carefully placed simple or running sutures (nonabsorbable) are also suitable. The use of pledgets (i.e. Teflon) may be particularly useful to support sutures during primary closure, or reimplantation of the diaphragm onto the lateral chest wall, if tissue loss has occured. Large diaphragmatic defects may occasionally require placement of a prosthesis (i.e. polytetrafluoroethylene (PTFE), polypropylene mesh) for reconstruction, with further soft tissue coverage available from regional muscle flaps.

Trauma

Injury to the diaphragm may present early or late following blunt or penetrating trauma, and may involve either hemidiaphragm. Therefore, a high index of suspicion is required, as many late presentations are simply the result of overlooked injuries.

1. Penetrating injuries. Knife or bullet injuries may result initially in more obvious wounds to the abdominal or thoracic viscera. Examination of the diaphragm at laparotomy (laparoscopy) or thoracotomy (thoracoscopy) is essential to avoid missing an injury. Primary repair of a diaphragmatic injury is required. Patients not undergoing exploration should be followed carefully.

2. Blunt injuries. Motor vehicle accidents, for example, may result in diaphragmatic rupture. Although injuries are reported predominantly on the left, right-sided injuries are now recognized with increased frequency. Herniation of abdominal viscera (i.e. spleen, stomach, colon, small intestine) is present in over 50% of patients, and may be suspected preoperatively by an abnormal CXR. Barium contrast studies, ultrasound or CT scanning may confirm the diagnosis. If surgery is required, the left hemidiaphragm is generally best explored through the abdomen and the right through the chest.

3. Late presentation. The late presentation of a diaphragmatic hernia is generally the result of a missed diaphragmatic injury. Symptoms may be quite nonspecific (i.e. abdominal or chest discomfort) or life-threatening, with acute intestinal obstruction. Surgery is required to reduce the hernia and close the defect. A thoracic approach (eighth or ninth interspace) is particularly useful in the presence of long-standing adhesions.

Tumors

1. Primary. These tumors are rare. The majority are of mesenchymal (connective tissue) origin. Fibrosarcoma is probably the most common malignant tumor. Symptoms may be quite nonspecific, and suspected tumors should be staged by CT scan. Surgical excision is recommended if possible for diagnosis and therapy. A wide margin of normal tissue is generally required to ensure a complete resection, and diaphragmatic reconstruction is frequently necessary.

2. Direct invasion. Direct invasion of thoracic (i.e. lung carcinoma) or abdominal tumors occurs not infrequently. When appropiate, an *en bloc* excision is advised.

3. Secondary. These tumors (i.e. metastases) of the diaphragm rarely occur as isolated metastases.

Diaphragmatic paralysis

Generally arises as a consequence of injury to the phrenic nerve.

- Cardiothoracic surgery, particularly reoperative or transplantation. Direct injury, traction injury, use of electrocautery or hypothermia are mechanisms of injury.
- Trauma; by deceleration, blast or blunt injury.
- Neuromuscular disorders.
- Infective; viral, bacterial, tuberculous, etc.
- Idiopathic.

In children, diaphragmatic paralysis may result is significant respiratory difficulty. Lung expansion appears to be limited as a result of mediastinal shift, relatively weak intercostal musculature and upward movement of abdominal viscera. By contrast, unilateral diaphragmatic paralysis in adults appears to produce relatively little respiratory difficulty, except when supine. Symptoms and abnormal pulmonary function studies (vital capacity, total lung capacity) may improve for up to 6 months following diagnosis, and are thought to be a consequence of accessory muscle use.

1. Management. Plication of the diaphragm has been used successfully in infants and adults, although the indications for this procedure are unclear. Plication appears to alter the configuration of the diaphragm, allowing total lung capacity, vital capacity, FEV_1 and diffusing capacity to increase. The duration of long-term improvement is unknown, but gradual deterioration of clinical and objective lung function has been reported after 5 years. Using a thoracic approach, the diaphragm is plicated using multiple, interrupted, buttressed sutures, until it becomes relatively taut.

Further reading

Graeber GM, Miller JI. The diaphragm. In: Pearson FG, Deslauriers J, Ginsberg RJ, Hiebert CA, McKneally MF, Urschel HC, eds. *Thoracic Surgery*. New York: Churchill Livingstone, 1995; 1305.

Related topics of interest

DIAPHRAGMATIC HERNIAE (CONGENITAL)

Gail Darling

The complex embryology of the diaphragm underlies the variety of congenital diaphragmatic defects that may arise from failure of development or fusion of the following embryonic components during week 8–10 of intrauterine life.

- Septum transversum, which forms the anterior and pericardial portions of the central tendon.
- Pleuroperitoneal membranes, paired structures forming the postero-lateral component.
- Dorsal esophageal mesentery, forming the posterior median element of the diaphragm (associated with the aorta, vena cava and esophagus).
- Body wall, comprising lateral muscle masses originating from the third to fifth cervical myotomes, which migrate caudally.

Bochdalek (postero–lateral) hernia

Failure of the pleuroperitoneal canal to close at 8 weeks' gestation allows the foregut to herniate into the chest cavity. Ipsilateral lung development is impaired, and the resulting pulmonary hypoplasia is the main cause of associated morbidity and mortality. Pulmonary hypoplasia leads to hypoxia, acidosis, pulmonary hypertension, reverse flow through the patent ductus and open foramen ovale, resulting in a right to left shunt and persistent fetal circulation. The contralateral lung may also be affected due to mediastinal shift. Forty percent of children have associated anomalies (cardiac, neural, renal, intestinal malrotation) and 30% have chromonsomal abnormalities (i.e. trisomy 18, 13).

1. Presentation. Patients present with respiratory distress, tracheal shift, absent breath sounds on the affected side, and a scaphoid abdomen. The severity of the symptoms depends on the degree of pulmonary compromise. A small hernia may present with feeding difficulties or be asymptomatic.

Diagnosis is established by a CXR, showing intestinal contents in the chest, usually on the left side.

2. Management. The following techniques are used in the management of Bochdalek hernia. (i) Intubation and mechanical ventilation (often with 100% oxygen, hyperventilation). Possible high-frequency ventilation or extracorporeal membrane oxygenation for infants who do not respond appropiately. (ii) Decompression of the stomach (using a nasogastric tube). (iii) Correction of acidosis by limiting fluids. (iv) Surgical repair when stable. The timing of surgery (i.e. immediate vs. delayed) is still controversial. Reduction of abdominal viscera, excision of the hernia sac (20% cases) and repair of the diaphragm are performed transabdominally. Large diaphragmatic defects may require a prosthesis. A temporary ventral hernia or silon pouch may be required to accommodate the reduced abdominal viscera without tension.

Postoperatively the chest tube is placed into an underwater seal without suction, to avoid pulmonary barotrauma. Pulmonary vasoconstriction may be precipitated by minor physiological changes, which should be avoided.

Mortality is high (>50%), especially in babies requiring urgent treatment within the first 24 hours of life. Chronic pulmonary disease and mental retardation may be present in survivors. Recent attempts have been made to correct this defect *in utero*.

Morgagni (retrosternal–anterior) hernia

A rare hernia, occuring between the xiphoid and costochondral attachments where the internal thoracic vessels penetrate the anterior diaphragm. Usually occurs on the right side, in adults, particularly females.

1. Presentation. This hernia is asymptomatic, and is usually discovered on an incidental CXR. There may be vague upper abdominal discomfort (i.e. pain, fullness).

Diagnosis is usually made on CXR, but may be interpreted as a large pericardial fat pad or pericardial cyst. Ultrasound, CT scanning, contrast gastrointestinal (GI) studies or a diagnostic pneumoperitoneum may be useful.

2. Management. Surgery is generally recommended, using an abdominal approach with a midline or subcostal incision. After reduction of the hernia contents and excision of the sac, the defect is closed by primary repair or patch.

Septum transversum hernia

Very rare herniation of the central diaphragm, associated with other midline congenital defects (i.e. omphalocele, sternal clefts, etc.). Herniation of the heart through the defect (absent pericardium) may occur. Surgical repair of the defect is required, and is best approached abdominally.

Eventration

Defined as an abnormal elevation of the diaphragm. The congenital form results from failure of muscularization of the fetal diaphragm, and is associated with prematurity, chromosomal abnormalities and congential malformations. The acquired form generally results from phrenic nerve injury.

1. Presentation
- *Neonates.* Respiratory distress, similiar to Bochdalek hernia if large.
- *Adults.* Generally asymptomatic (40–50%). Symptoms may be nonspecific, or may include dyspnoea, dysphagia, reflux.

Diagnosis is made by CXR, and confirmed by fluroscopy (sniff test) which demonstrates paradoxical movement of the affected side, or ultrasound of the diaphragm.

2. *Management.* Depends on the severity of the symptoms in adults. In children, ventilator dependency, repeated lung infections, feeding difficulties, failure to thrive or a large eventration in an asymptomatic child (which may interfere with lung development), are indications for surgery. Surgical repair comprises plication of the diaphragm.

Further reading

Graeber GM, Davtyan J, Miller JI. Congenital hernias. In: Pearson FG, Deslauriers J, Ginsberg RJ, Hiebert CA, McKneally MF, Urschel HC, eds. *Thoracic Surgery*. New York: Churchill Livingstone, 1995; 1313.

Related topics of interest

DIAPHRAGMATIC PACING

Alan G. Casson

Diaphragmatic pacing by phrenic nerve stimulation entered clinical practice following the development of modern pacemaker technology, and has been used successfully in a limited number of centers for treating ventilatory insufficiency in selected patients.

Etiology and indications

1. Quadraplegia. Usually resulting from trauma (partial or complete) to the spinal cord (or brainstem) above C6. May also occur as a result of tumor invasion, therapy (i.e. radiation, surgery), infarction, neuromuscular (i.e. syringomyelia) or other demyelinating diseases.

2. Respiratory diseases. Idiopathic central alveolar hypoventilation, chronic obstructive lung disease (relative).

Requirements for phrenic nerve pacing

- Artificial ventilation (>1 month) for respiratory paralysis. A backup positive pressure ventilator must always be available.
- Intact phrenic nerve (lower motor neurones).
- Objective response of the diaphragm to transcutaneous phrenic nerve stimulation.
- Normal cerebral function, compliance and family support.
- Satisfactory pulmonary function studies and arterial blood gases. A permanent tracheostomy is required.
- Acceptable surgical/anesthetic risk.

Contraindications

- Nonviable phrenic nerves.
- Progressive neurological disease (or tumor).
- Primary diaphragmatic disease (i.e. myopathy).
- Severe intrinsic pulmonary disease.

Surgery

1. Cervical. The phrenic nerve is identified on the anterior scalene muscle within the scalene triangle. The electrode is implanted into the muscle below the nerve and tunneled over the clavicle to a subcutaneous anterior chest-wall pocket containing the pacemaker receiver.

2. Thoracic. A second or third interspace incision is made anteriorly and the phrenic nerve identified on the pericardium below the junction of the SVC and atrium (right side) or at the level of the superior pulmonary vein (left side). The electrode is placed adjacent to the neurovascular bundle and tunneled to the receiver. The pacing threshold is then set to a minimum to achieve diaphragmatic excursion between 80 and 85%, assessed using fluoroscopy or ultrasound. Pacing is generally started 2 weeks postoperatively (to allow postoperative edema to settle), and for no more than 12 hours daily (to avoid diaphragmatic fatigue).

Further reading

Glenn WL, Phelps ML, Elefteriades JA. Twenty years of experience in phrenic nerve stimulation to pace the diaphragm. *Pace*, 1986; **9:** 789.

Marcy TW, Oloke JS. Diaphragm pacing for ventilatory insufficiency. *Journal of Intensive Care Medicine*, 1987; **2:** 345.

Related topic of interest

Diaphragm (p. 66)

EMPYEMA

Chris Compeau, Michael R. Johnston

A thoracic empyema is defined as pus in the pleural space, which may be localized or involve the entire pleural space. Successful therapy depends on a clear understanding of the pathogenesis of empyema. This frequently requires considerable clinical judgement and experience, particularly as many patients will be at high risk from coexisting disease (i.e. chronic lung diseases, diabetes mellitus, malignancy, etc.), immunosuppression, nutritional deficiency, etc. Prompt intervention to adequately drain and obliterate the infected space is essential, but the timing and type of drainage procedure depends on several factors. The recent resurgence of tuberculosis and increasing frequency of anaerobic, mixed and drug-resistant microorganisms, suggests that pleural-space infections will continue to challenge the thoracic surgeon. Postpneumonectomy empyema and bronchopleural fistula remain a particular challenge to treat.

Etiology

The pleural space, particularly when it contains fluid or blood, may become infected by (i) direct inoculation at surgery or by penetrating chest injuries, or (ii) by contamination from contiguous sources. The commonest cause is bronchopulmonary infection, with direct spread across pleura or rupture of peripheral microabscesses resulting in a parapneumonic effusion. Rupture of a lung abscess, mediastinal abscess (secondary to esophageal perforation), or transdiaphragmatic spread from a subphrenic abscess, are occasionally causative. Hematogenous spread from distant sites may occur but is uncommon.

Microbiology

In the pre-antibiotic era, the predominant microorganisms were pneumococci and *Streptococcus pneumoniae*. Increasing antibiotic use was not only associated with a reduction in the incidence and mortality of empyema, but a change in the spectrum of microorganisms. Mixed infections (generally three species) are found commonly today, with the following microorganisms isolated frequently:

1. Aerobic organisms
- *Gram-positive. Streptococcus, Staphylococcus (Staphylococcus aureus* in childern).
- *Gram-negative.* Coliforms, *Proteus, H. influenzae* (children).

2. Anaerobic organisms. Most common in adults, related to aspiration, and include *Bacteroides, Fusobacterium* and *Peptostreptococcus* (mouth organisms). Increasingly, culture of pleural/empyema fluid will not establish a microbiologic diagnosis. This is most often the result of previous treatment with antibiotics, or improper culture of anaerobic organisms.

Pathogenesis

The American Thoracic Society (1962) divided the evolution of parapneumonic effusions into empyemas into three stages, usually occuring over 3–6 weeks.

1. Exudative stage. An outpouring of thin pleural fluid occurs in response to pleural inflammation. Fibrin is deposited over the pleural surfaces, but is not thick, and if the pleural space is drained, the underlying lung will re-expand.

2. Fibrinopurulent stage. Bacterial invasion of pleural fluid and an influx of polymorphs, result in the pleural fluid becoming turbid and purulent. Heavy fibrin deposition on the visceral and parietal pleura may prevent lung re-expansion and loculations may be present.

3. Organization stage. Pus is very thick. Ingrowth of fibroblasts results in collagen formation; the lung is trapped in a thick fibrous peel.

Complications of an untreated empyema are:

- Pulmonary fibrosis and contraction of the chest cavity.
- Spontaneous drainage of pus through the chest wall (empyema necessitatis) or through the bronchial tree (bronchopleural fistula).
- Distant infection of bone (osteomyelitis), or local spread to the pericardium or mediastinum.

Diagnosis

1. Clinical/radiological
- Chest pain, purulent sputum, fever, leukocytosis.
- CXR showing a pleural effusion.
- CT scanning will differentiate a pleural collection from a lung abscess, define loculations, thickness of the pleural peel and demonstrate coexisting thoracic disease. It is a useful study for planning surgery.
- Ultrasound may also be useful to define pleural collections (especially in relation to the diaphragm), and prior to percutaneous drainage procedures.

2. Thoracentesis
- Pus (gross appearance and odor).
- *Microbiology.* Send pleural fluid (and sputum) for Gram stain, culture (aerobic and anaerobic) and sensitivity.
- *Biochemistry.* Several parameters and formulae (some quite complex) have been proposed to differentiate empyemas from contaminated pleural effusions, and as a guide to therapy. These remain controversial, but the following suggest empyema:

  (a) High protein (i.e. exudate, >30 mg/dl).
  (b) Low pH (<7.2).

(c) High LDH (>1000 IU/l).

(d) Low glucose (<50 mg/dl).

Treatment

1. General. Supportive respiratory care, physiotherapy, fluids and nutrition. Treat associated medical conditions and the underlying cause of the empyema.

2. Antibiotics. Appropiate selection of systemic antibiotic therapy directed by Gram stain and culture.

3. Surgery. Intercostal tube drainage [using a large diameter (>34 F) tube] may be curative if performed early enough for a parapneumonic effusion/Stage I acute empyema, provided complete drainage and obliteration of the pleural space is achieved. Tubes are connected to underwater seal drainage (closed drainage) and suction initially. A tube can be removed safely provided there is no air leak, when the daily drainage is less than 100 ml, or is sterile. Otherwise, it may be converted to open tube drainage ('empyema tube') by cutting just beyond the skin edge. The tube is then progressively withdrawn several cm each week until it is completely removed from the chest.

Attempts at instilling fibrinolytic enzymes (i.e. streptokinase or urokinase) have received increasing attention, especially using CT- or ultrasound-guided catheter insertion (interventional radiology). The indications for this approach are controversial, but patient selection appears to be key to a successful outcome.

In modern practice, early surgical drainage may be performed safely, with reduced hospitalization. Use of a mini-thoracotomy, pleuroscopy or VATS is highly effective in selected patients.

Open window thoracostomy (modified Eloesser flap) is effective for prolonged drainage of an empyema cavity. The thoracostomy should be placed in a dependent position and should be sufficiently large (at least two ribs resected; suture skin to pleura) to prevent premature closure. If performed early in the disease process, packing is usually required initially to debride the cavity, stabilize the mediastinum or control a bronchopleural fistula. Closure of the thoracostomy is best accomplished by muscle transposition or thoracoplasty. Sterilization of the space by instillation of antibiotic solution prior to closure of the thoracostomy (Claggett procedure) is associated with a high (50%) failure rate.

Decortication to remove an empyema and the constricting pleural peel, may be performed acutely (especially if early pleuroscopy or VATS debridement fails) or as a delayed procedure (traditional approach). A posterolateral thoracotomy is employed for access; the empyema cavity is debrided, and the trapped underlying lung mobilized and re-expanded. Multiple chest tubes may be placed postoperatively to control any air leak from the raw lung surface and to facilitate re-expansion of the underlying lung.

Further reading

American Thoracic Society. Management of non tuberculous empyema. *American Review of Respiratory Disease*, 1962; **85:** 935.

Gregoire R, Deslauriers J, Beaulieu M, Piraux M. Thoracoplasty: its forgotten role in the management of non tuberculous post pneumonectomy empyema. *Canadian Journal of Surgery*, 1987; **30:** 343.

Houston MC. Pleural fluid pH: diagnostic, therapeutic and prognostic value. *American Journal of Surgery*, 1987; 154: 333.

Lawrence DR, Ohri SK, Moxon RE, Townsend ER, Fountain SW. Thoracoscopic debridement of empyema thoracis. *Annals of Thoracic Surgery*, 1997; **64:** 1448.

Miller JI, ed. Empyema, spaces and fistula. *Chest Surgery Clinics of North America*, 1996; **6:** 403.

Orringer MB. Thoracic empyema – back to basics. *Chest*, 1988; **93:** 901.

Related topics of interest

Bronchopleural fistula (p. 29)
Chest tubes (p. 42)

ESOPHAGEAL ATRESIA AND CONGENITAL ANOMALIES

Donna E. Maziak, F. Griff Pearson

Congenital anomalies of the foregut are uncommon. The precise cause and developmental alterations responsible for these defects are still not known with certainty. This chapter will review briefly the key features associated with the most frequent disorders: esophageal atresia and tracheoesophageal fistula, esophageal cysts/duplications, congenital stenosis and webs, diverticulae and vascular rings.

Esophageal atresia and tracheoesophageal fistula

1. Embryology. When the embryo is approximately 4 weeks, a small diverticulum appears at the ventral wall of the foregut. This respiratory diverticulum is gradually separated from the dorsal part of the foregut through a partition. The foregut is divided into a ventral portion, the respiratory primordium and a distal portion, the esophagus. Any interruption of the elongation and partitioning of the esophageal and tracheal tubes is thought to lead to a persistent fistula and atresia, with a wide range of defects. The incidence of these anomalies is about 1 in 4000 births.

2. Classification. The classification given in *Table 1* (Gross, 1953) is widely used today.

3. Clinical presentation. The diagnosis is suspected by a maternal history of polyhydramnios, and by the following signs after birth: regurgitation of saliva or of the first feed, aspiration during feeding followed by choking and coughing, abdominal distention and chemical pneumonitis. A differential diagnosis of recurrent pneumonia in the neonate includes cystic fibrosis, agammaglobulinemia, congenital hiatus hernia, esophageal stenosis, tracheal compression by vascular rings, traumatic or neurogenic dysfunction of the esophagus. The inability to pass a catheter (i.e. feeding tube) into the stomach, and radiologic contrast studies will confirm the diagnosis. Associated congenital anomalies occur in 20% of patients: the combination of vertebral defects (23%), imperforate anus

Table 1. Classification of esophageal atresia

Type	Description
A	Pure esophageal atresia (8%)
B	Esophageal atresia with upper pouch fistula to the trachea (1%)
C	Esophageal atresia with lower pouch fistula to the trachea (86%)
D	Esophageal atresia with lower and upper fistulae (1%)
E	Fistula without atresia (4%)

(10%), tracheoesophageal fistula, radial and renal dysplasia (7%) (VATER) is recognized, particularly in infants weighing less than 2 kg. Mortality is higher with the VATER association.

4. Management. Treatment of these infants is started immediately once the diagnosis is confirmed: treatment comprises 30° head-up position, intravenous fluids, antibiotic therapy (even if pneumonia is not yet clinically present), and suction/aspiration of the upper pouch. Definitive management is dictated by risk as outlined in the risk classification below (*Table 2*) (Waterson, 1962).

5. Operative technique
- Transthoracic approach: transpleural, extrapleural.
- Careful dissection to minimize vagal injury and vascular supply, especially to the lower esophageal segment, and during dissection of the upper esophageal segment from the posterior membranous trachea.
- The fistula is localized, divided or sutured, and healthy tissues interposed.
- A single-layer tension-free anastomosis is performed for defects <2 cm. For long gaps, additional length may be obtained by esophageal myotomy.
- Esophageal replacement using colon, gastric tubes, stomach or jejunum may be required.
- A gastrostomy is used if surgery is delayed. Its routine use at the time of definitive surgery is controversial.

6. Results. Associated congenital anomalies account for the majority of early deaths, with variable mortality rates from 5 to 15%. Postoperative morbidity results from anastomotic leaks, gastroesophageal reflux, stricture, recurrent tracheoesophageal fistula and tracheomalacia. Long-term functional problems are common, and include motility disorders (possibly neurologic), gastroesophageal reflux, late strictures and post-thoracotomy chest-wall deformity (i.e. elevated shoulder, underdeveloped

Table 2. Risk classification for esophageal atresia

Class	Condition	Treatment
A	>2500 g and well	Surgery with primary reconstruction
B	(1) 1800–2500 g and well (2) >2500 g with moderate pneumonia and other congenital anomalies	Initially nonoperative (antibiotics and gastrostomy), surgery when stable
C	(1) <1800 g (2) >1800 g with severe pneumonia and severe congenital anomalies	Divide the fistula; and staged surgery

hemithorax, scoliosis). Late problems following esophageal substitutions relate to the intrinsic problems of the interposed organ.

Esophageal cysts/duplications

Esophageal cysts are rare lesions, usually referred to as duplications. They are found in a wide variety of locations, with differing histology and possible embrologic origin. Duplications are usually smooth cystic masses distinct from the esophagus but attached to it by a common wall. No communication to the lumen is found. Cysts in the posterior mediastinum are believed to be of neuroenteric origin and from incomplete separation of the notochord and foregut (i.e. part of the split notochord syndrome). The cellular composition is variable and may be used to determine the embryological origin: cartilage, squamous epithelium or gastric mucosa.

Patients may present with respiratory symptoms, dysphagia related to esophageal compression or be asymptomatic, the cyst being detected on a routine CXR. Diagnosis includes CXR, barium swallow, CT and possibly MRI if spinal involvement is suspected.

The natural history of these cyts is variable and includes: a mass effect on surrounding structures (i.e. lung, heart, esophagus) due to increasing size; acute medistinitis from cyst rupture; and anemia or bleeding from peptic ulceration. Although they are considered to be benign lesions, malignant degeneration is reported and surgical resection is recommended.

Congenital stenosis and webs

These are rare malformations of the esophagus with an incidence of 1 in 25 000–50 000 births. They are thought to arise by the following mechanisms: (i) Segmental fibromuscular hypertrophy (usually distal esophagus). (ii) Intramural rests of tracheobronchial tissue (usually distal esophagus). (iii) Membranous webs (anywhere).

The degree of stenosis and the location will determine the symptoms. Quite often diagnosis is delayed until solids are introduced into the diet. With the delay, marked proximal dilatation and dysmotility of the esophagus may have developed. Diagnosis is made by radiologic contrast study and esophagoscopy. Esophageal dilatation provides effective treatment in the majority of patients, although surgical resection and reconstruction may be indicated for thicker, lower esophageal stenoses resulting from tracheobronchial remnants.

Congenital esophageal diverticulum

These rare abnormalities; can occur anywhere along the esophagus. This is a true diverticulum; believed to result from persistence of a diverticulum that occurs during formation of the foregut. Clinical symptoms vary depending on the size and location, and diagnosis is by barium swallow and esophagogastroscopy. The preferred method of therapy is resection. The esophageal mucosa should be closed in a transverse direction to minimize the possibility of recurrence or stricture.

Vascular rings Vascular rings result from abnormal development of the embryonic aortic arch. The most common anomalies resulting in rings are: double aortic arch (most frequent), right aortic arch with left ligamentum arteriosum, left aortic arch and pulmonary artery sling. Compression of the trachea and esophagus result in varying degrees of dysphagia and airway obstruction. Diagnosis is by barium swallow, bronchoscopy, chest CT and occasionally angiography. Patients are managed by surgical correction of the vascular anomaly.

Further reading

Ashcraft KW. Esophageal atresia and tracheoesophageal fistula. *Chest Surgery Clinics of North America*, 1993; **3:** 4777.

Gross RE. *Surgery of Infancy and Childhood*. Philadelphia: W.B. Saunders, 1953.

Tsai JY, Berkery L, Wesson DE, Redo SF, Spigland NA. Esophageal atresia and tracheoesophageal fistula: surgical experience over two decades. *Annals of Thoracic Surgery*, 1997; **64:** 778.

Waterson DJ, Carter REB, Aberden E. Oesophageal atreasia: tracheoesophageal fistula: a study of survival in 218 infants. *Lancet*, 1962; **i:** 819.

Related topic of interest

Congenital bronchopulmonary anomalies (p. 56)

ESOPHAGEAL CANCER: DIAGNOSIS AND STAGING

Renee Kennedy, Alan G. Casson

As benign and malignant esophageal diseases often present clinically with dysphagia, it is essential to obtain a definitive tissue diagnosis of malignancy to guide further investigations and treatment. Currently, the stage of an esophageal carcinoma is the best predictor of survival. However, the relative inaccessibility of the esophagus to preoperative investigation, inconsistent correlation between preoperative imaging and operative findings, and the lack of a totally satisfactory tumor node metastasis (TNM) system, have limited consistent preoperative staging of this disease.

Clinical presentation

Symptoms and signs generally arise as a result of local invasion of the primary tumor, or from distant metastases.

1. Primary tumor. Dysphagia is the most common presenting symptom, being reported by over 90% of patients. Other symptoms suggesting esophageal obstruction or dysfunction (i.e. general difficulty or a change in swallowing, regurgitation or vomiting, odynophagia) are common, but nonspecific. Pain (epigastric, back, neck) is an uncommon presenting symptom (<20% of patients), and may arise from local tumor infiltration, esophagitis, metastasis to intra-abdominal lymph nodes or bone. Respiratory symptoms, especially cough after swallowing, suggest aspiration or an esophagotracheal or -bronchial fistula.

Patients with Barrett's esophagus, in endoscopic surveillance programs, may have symptoms of associated gastroesophageal reflux or may be asymptomatic.

2. Distant metastases. At least 50% of patients will have evidence of systemic disease at presentation. General symptoms, including weight loss and cachexia, are reported by over 50% of patients. The most common sites of metastatic disease are lung (30–50%) and liver (20–50%), but other sites (i.e. bone, adrenal, kidney, abdominal lymph nodes, etc.) are increasingly recognized.

Diagnosis

1. Physical examination. Look for enlarged cervical or supraclavicular lymph nodes, signs of chronic aspiration (rales, rhonchi, consolidation), upper abdominal mass, hepatomegaly, generalized wasting.

2. Laboratory investigations. These are nonspecific and may include anemia, hypoproteinemia, abnormal liver function tests or hypercalcemia.

3. Chest X-ray. CXR may demonstrate pulmonary metastases, pulmonary infiltrates or pneumonia, a soft-tissue mass or an air/fluid level in the mediastinum.

4. Barium esophagram. This should be obtained as the initial investigation (prior to instrumentation) in patients with suspected esophageal cancer. Defines foregut anatomy, in addition to the level and extent of esophageal obstruction. Use of dilute barium is preferred, especially if there is a possibility of aspiration or a malignant esophagotracheal or -bronchial fistula.

5. Esophagogastroscopy. This investigation is performed under local anesthesia, using flexible fiberoptic instrumentation. Alternatively, the rigid esophagoscope may be used under general anesthesia. The site and extent (i.e. measurements) of the esophageal tumor are evaluated endoscopically. The relationship to the esophagogastric junction and cricopharyngeus is also noted, along with other mucosal abnormalities (i.e. Barrett's esophagus). Multiple biopsies of the tumor are taken to obtain a histologic diagnosis, and obstructing tumors may be dilated (or stented) during this procedure. The stomach is evaluated for potential reconstruction of the upper gastrointestinal tract, and to exclude gastric disease (i.e. peptic ulceration, gastric tumors).

6. Computed tomography. CT scanning of the primary tumor may underestimate the extent of local disease or the invasion of adjacent structures. Overall accuracy is reported to be between 60 and 90%, but may be improved with the use of intravenous contrast, high-resolution scanning or with the development of new generations of scanners. The significance of enlarged lymph nodes (mediastinal, upper abdominal) is controversial. Nodes larger than 10 mm in transverse diameter are considered radiologically to be positive for metastasis. Accuracy rates of CT scanning for nodal metastases are generally low (50–60%), as nodes may be enlarged for other reasons (i.e. infection, sarcoidosis, etc.), and small nodes may have microscopic metastases. A histologic diagnosis is essential to diagnose lymph node metastasis. CT scanning of potential distant metastatic sites (i.e. brain) is performed selectively. Lung and liver are routinely imaged on the chest CT.

7. Endoscopic ultrasound. The depth of tumor penetration (all T stages) is currently most accurately (80–95%) assessed preoperatively using endoscopic ultrasound. This technique may also be used to assess periesophageal lymph-node metastasis, but with less accuracy. Endoscopic ultrasound is currently useful only as a research tool in non-obstructing tumors, but future advances in ultrasound technology are likely to increase the clinical application of this technique for pre-operative staging.

8. Bronchoscopy. This should always be performed for tumors of the upper esophagus (i.e. at or above the carina, in close proximity to the airway), or if a malignant fistula is suspected. It is also useful in obstructing lesions at all levels for bronchial toilet and to obtain appropriate samples for culture and sensitivity.

9. Additional studies. MRI currently has little advantage over CT scanning for intrathoracic staging of esophageal cancer. Recent reports of positron emission tomography (PET) scanning are encouraging, but this technique is not widely available. Minimally invasive techniques (i.e. laparoscopy and thoracoscopy) are currently under investigation as invasive staging procedures for esophageal cancers. Aortography, azygography, gallium scanning and lymphoscintigraphy have all been utilized for staging esophageal cancers, but have not been adopted into routine clinical practice.

Staging

The stage of an esophageal carcinoma may be determined clinically (i.e. preoperatively), at surgery or pathologically. Pathologic stage currently provides the most accurate prognostic information. One area of particular controversy is staging of adenocarcinomas at the esophagogastric junction. Tumors believed to be of primary esophageal origin (see 'Esophageal cancer: etiology and pathology', p. 88) should be staged as esophageal carcinomas, whereas tumors of gastric origin (including cardia) should be staged as gastric carcinomas.

1. T descriptor
- Tis. Carcinoma *in situ.*
- T1. Tumor invades lamina propria, muscularis mucosa or submucosa, but does not extend into the muscularis propria.
- T2. Tumor invades muscularis propria.
- T3. Tumor extends beyond the muscularis propria into the periesophageal tissues.
- T4. Tumor invades adjacent structures.

2. N descriptor
- N0. No regional lymph-node metastasis.
- N1. Regional lymph-node metastasis.

Regional lymph nodes are difficult to define and depend on the anatomic level of the tumor. Furthermore, attempts at lymph-node mapping (similar to lung cancer) have not been widely adopted for esophageal cancer. In general, lower thoracic lymph node metastases from a cervical esophageal tumor are considered distant (M) disease, as are celiac lymph node metastases from a lower-third esophageal carcinoma.

3. M descriptor
- No distant metastases.
- Distant metastases.

For tumors of lower thoracic esophagus:

- M1a. Metastasis in coeliac lymph nodes.
- M1b. Other distant metastasis.

For tumors of upper thoracic esophagus:

- M1a. Metastasis in cervical lymph nodes.
- M1b. Other distant metastasis.

For tumors of mid-thoracic esophagus:

- M1a. Not applicable.
- M1b. Nonregional lymph node or other distant metastasis.

Stage groupings – TNM subsets

Table 1 gives the corresponding TNM subsets for each stage of esophageal cancer.

Table 1. TNM subsets for the stages of esophageal cancer

Stage	TNM subsets		
0	Tis	N0	M0
I	T1	N0	M0
IIA	T2	N0	M0
	T3	N0	M0
IIB	T1	N1	M0
	T2	N1	M0
III	T3	N1	M0
	T4	Any N	M0
IV	Any T	Any N	M1
IVA	Any T	Any N	M1a
IVB	Any T	Any N	M1b

Significance of staging

In node negative (N0) patients (without distant metastases: M0), the depth of the primary tumor has prognostic value, with 5-year survival rates ranging from 75–85% (T1) to below 25% (T3).

Survival of patients with regional lymph node metastases (N1), but without distant disease (M0) is independent of T-stage (although fewer early T-stage tumors will be found with nodal metastases overall). Five-year survival for patients with N1 M0 disease is <10%, whereas it is >25% for patients with N0 M0 disease. Patients with 1–3 positive (N1) nodes have intermediate survival (10–15% at 5 years).

The presence of distant metastases significantly reduces survival, with only occasional patients surviving 5 years.

Further reading

Casson AG. Staging. In: Pearson FG, Deslauriers J, Ginsberg RJ, Hiebert CA, McKneally MF, Urschel HC, eds. *Esophageal Surgery*. New York: Churchill Livingstone, 1995; 560.

Farrow DC, Vaughan TL. Determinants of survival following the diagnosis of esophageal adenocarcinoma (United States). *Cancer Causes and Control*, 1996; **7:** 322.

Holscher AH, Siewert JR. Classification of adenocarcinomas of the esophagogastric junction. In: Peracchia A, Rosati R, Bonavina L, Fumagalli U, Bona S, Chella B, eds. *Recent Advances in Diseases of the Esophagus*. Bologna: Monduzzi Editore, 1996; 549.

Krasna MJ. Thoracoscopic staging of esophageal carcinoma. *Chest Surgery Clinics of North America*, 1995; **5:** 489.

Luketich JD, Schauer PR, Meltzer CC, Landrenau RJ, Urso GK, Townsend DW, Ferson PF, Keenan RJ, Belani CP. Role of positron emission tomography in staging esophageal cancer. *Annals of Thoracic Surgery*, 1997; **64:** 765.

Siewert JR, Holscher AH, Dittler HJ. Preoperative staging and risk analysis in esophageal carcinoma. *Hepato-gastroenterology* 1990; **37:** 382.

Stein HJ. Esophageal cancer: screening and surveillance. *Diseases of the Esophagus*, 1996; **9 (Suppl 1):** 3.

Related topics of interest

Barrett's esophagus (p. 16)
Esophageal cancer: etiology and pathology (p. 88)
Esophagoscopy, dilation and stenting (p. 113)

ESOPHAGEAL CANCER: ETIOLOGY AND PATHOLOGY

Renee Kennedy, Alan G. Casson

Squamous cell carcinoma of the esophagus is one of the most frequent malignancies world-wide. Epidemiologic studies from North America and Europe recently confirmed clinical suspicions that primary adenocarcinomas of the lower esophagus and esophagogastric junction are being seen more frequently. The rise in the rate of incidence of esophageal adenocarcinomas has exceeded that of any other solid tumor over the past two decades. The factors underlying this change are unknown.

Etiology

Epidemiology

The disease is characterized by striking geographical variation in incidence between countries and within distinct geographic regions. High-incidence areas are China, South Africa, northern Iran, temperate South America and northern France. Low-incidence areas include northern Africa, central America, western Asia and Polynesia. Such geographic variations in incidence suggest a predominant role for environmental factors in the etiology of esophageal cancer. A rising incidence of primary esophageal adenocarcinomas has been reported in North America. Between 1976 and 1987 the average annual rate of increase was 9.4% for white males. Similar trends were reported in Europe. Interestingly, while overall rates of gastric cancer declined over the same time, gastric cardia cancers increased at a 4.3% annual rate.

Age, sex, race

The highest mortality rates are generally reported for males aged between 60 and 70 years, and the disease is seen infrequently below age 40 years. Males are generally affected more frequently than females, but the sex ratio narrows in high-incidence regions. Racial and ethnic differences are reported in high-incidence areas, but the significance of this observation is unknown. In the United States, the black population appears to be at increased risk for developing esophageal squamous cell carcinomas, whereas adenocarcinomas predominate among white males.

Diet

Dietary and nutritional factors have been consistently implicated in the etiology of esophageal cancer. In general, populations living in high-incidence regions have been shown to have poor diet, often with specific nutritional deficiencies, or to be exposed to dietary carcinogens. Diets deficient in green vegetables, fruit, vitamins, trace elements or minerals have been consistently implicated. Dietary intervention studies, supplementing high-risk populations with multiple vitamins and minerals in an attempt to prevent esophageal carcinogenesis, are ongoing. Dietary carcinogens include nitrosamines and their precursors (nitrates and nitrites), frequently associated with an intake of pickled vegetables, cured meats or fish and the fungal contamination of ingested foods. Epidemiologic observations have been reproduced in laboratory studies using animal models.

Smoking and alcohol

A heavy alcohol intake, particularly in developed countries, has been associated with an increased incidence of squamous cell carcinoma. Recent studies suggest that this may not be as significant a factor for the development of esophageal adenocarcinomas. Statistically, there is a five- to sixfold increased risk of squamous cell carcinomas among cigarette smokers. The relationship between smoking and esophageal adenocarcinomas is less clear. An increased relative risk (exceeding 100-fold) of developing esophageal squamous cell carcinoma is seen when cigarette smoking is combined with heavy alcohol consumption. Local habits (i.e. chewing opium, betel or pipe tobacco residue) may account for an increased incidence of esophageal cancers in other high-incidence areas where cigarette smoking is uncommon.

Intrinsic esophageal disease

Various intrinsic diseases of the esophagus are associated with esophageal cancer, although patient numbers are small and statistical correlation is difficult.

1. Barrett's esophagus. See 'Barrett's esophagus', p. 16. Patients with a columnar-epithelium-lined esophagus (Barrett's esophagus) are estimated to be at least 30–40 times at increased risk of developing an esophageal adenocarcinoma than the general population.

2. Plummer–Vinson (Patterson–Kelly) syndrome. Atrophy of the oropharyngeal and esophageal mucosa, secondary to iron and vitamin (nicotinamide and lactoflavin) deficiency, is a risk factor for developing upper aerodigestive tract tumors. Dietary correction of these nutritional deficiencies has been shown to reduce the risk.

3. Achalasia. Squamous cell carcinomas have been shown to develop as an infrequent, late complication of untreated achalasia. Stasis, resulting in prolonged mucosal exposure to ingested carcinogens, has been proposed as a possible predisposing factor.

4. Corrosive injury. Occasional reports suggest that esophageal cancers may develop as a late complication of acid- or alkali-induced esophageal mucosal injury or stricture.

5. *Miscellaneous conditions*. Esophageal mucosal injury, resulting from the ingestion of hot liquids and solids, has been associated with esophageal cancer development in China, Uruguay, Brazil, Thailand and Iran. Reports of increased risk secondary to radiation injury, asbestos and rubber exposure, are infrequent.

Inheritance

The possibility that genetic factors might predispose to the development of esophageal cancer arose initially from two unrelated observations: an association with tylosis, and the occasional familial incidence or clustering of the disease. Tylosis is a rare familial (autosomal dominant) syndrome, characterized by thickening (hyperkeratosis) of the skin of the soles of the feet and palms of the hands. About 40% of family members develop esophageal squamous cell carcinoma by their mid-40s. Although familial clusterings of the disease may suggest exposure to common environmental factors, recent analysis of high-risk families in China suggested an autosomal recessive Mendelian inheritance for esophageal squamous cell carcinomas. Slight associations are also reported between esophageal cancer and blood group A, HLA A_2 and B_{40}.

Molecular genetic alterations

Molecular genetic alterations (i.e. *p53*, *erbB-1*, *myc*) have recently been reported in esophageal cancers and in premalignant Barrett's mucosa. The relative importance of individual genetic lesions, the sequence of genetic events, and the pathways by which oncogenes and tumor-suppressor genes modulate multistep esophageal tumorigenesis, are unknown.

Pathology

Squamous cell carcinoma

This remains the most common histologic subtype worldwide, accounting for over 80% of all primary esophageal cancers. Series from North American and European centers report a variable prevalence of esophageal squamous cell carcinomas, ranging from 40 to 60%.

The distribution of tumors along the esophagus is as follows: mid-third (50%), lower-third (30–40%), upper-third (10–20%). Macroscopic types are fungating, ulcerating, infiltrating and polypoid. Local invasion of the tumor is common, resulting in esophageal obstruction or direct invasion of neighboring structures (i.e. trachea, pericardium, aorta, etc.). Histologically, well-differentiated carcinomas have prominent keratinization, whereas poorly differentiated tumors display minimal keratinization. Grade, neural and vascular invasion are uncertain prognostic indicators.

Submucosal tumor spread (contiguous) proximally is frequently seen. Tumor will be found at 10 cm from the main tumor in <6% of cases. Metastasis to regional lymph nodes is seen in more than 50% of patients at diagnosis, and is a major determinant of survival. Lymph-node metastasis is now regarded as a marker of systemic disease. Lung (30–50%) and liver (20–50%) are the most frequent sites of distant metastasis.

Several distinct variants of squamous cell carcinoma have been described:

1. *Superficial.* The concept of superficially invasive (or early) esophageal squamous cell carcinoma arose from the Japanese and Chinese literature, reflecting early detection through screening programs. There is no consensus on a precise definition, although most investigators limit its use to an invasive tumor with local invasion not beyond the submucosa (T1).

2. *Basaloid.* Previously reported as adenoid cystic carcinomas, similar to basaloid lesions originating in the head and neck region. Characterized histologically by pleomorphic, closely packed basaloid cells (thought to be the cell of origin), forming lobules. Tumors have a similar appearance and outcome to the usual squamous cell carcinoma.

3. *Verrucous.* Similar to verrucous lesions of the oropharynx. Associated with heavy smoking, intrinsic esophageal diseases (i.e. achalasia, corrosive injury), and predominantly localized to the upper esophagus. Characterized by a less aggressive clinical course and rarely metastasizes.

4. *Adenosquamous carcinoma.* Basic appearance is a squamous cell carcinoma, with occasional intermixed focal glandular elements. Different from collision tumors where two distinct patterns of squamous cell and glandular differentiation meet with a distinct, pushing interface.

Adenocarcinoma

Primary adenocarcinomas of the esophagus account for up to 40% of tumors in recent series from several North American and European centers. They should be distinguished from adenocarcinomas of gastric origin (i.e. cardia, fundus).

Suggested clinicopathologic criteria, determined by endoscopy, radiology, at surgery or on pathologic examination, include:

- An associated Barrett's epithelium.
- Greater than 75% of the tumor mass involving the body of the tubular esophagus.
- Direct histologic invasion of periesophageal tissues.

- Minimal gastric involvement.
- Clinical symptoms of esophageal obstruction (i.e. dysphagia).

Uncommon esophageal malignancies

These account for less than 5% of all primary esophageal carcinomas.

Classification
- Undifferentiated carcinoma.
- Small cell carcinoma.
- Carcinoid.
- Malignant melanoma.
- Carcinosarcoma.
- Sarcomas (leiomyosarcoma, fibrosarcoma, liposarcoma, etc.).
- Malignant lymphoreticular disorders (i.e. Hodgkin's disease, plasmacytoma).
- Choriocarcinoma.
- Collision tumors.
- Secondary (metastatic) tumors.

Further reading

Begin LR. The pathobiology of esophageal cancer. In: Roth JA, Ruckdeschel JC, Weisenburger TH, eds. *Thoracic Oncology*, 2nd edn. Philadelphia: WB Saunders, 1995; 288.

Casson AG. Biology. In: Pearson FG, Deslauriers J, Ginsberg RJ, Hiebert CA, McKneally MF, Urschel HC, eds. *Esophageal Surgery*. New York: Churchill Livingstone, 1995; 539.

Chow WH, Finkle WD, McLaughlin JK, Frankl H, Ziel HK, Fraumeni JF. The relation of gastroesophageal reflux disease and its treatment to adenocarcinomas of the esophagus and gastric cardia. *Journal of the American Medical Association*, 1995; **274:** 474.

Haggitt RC. Adenocarcinoma in Barrett's esophagus: a new epidemic? *Human Pathology*, 1992; **23:** 475.

Lieberman MD, Franceschi D, Marsan B, Burt M. Esophageal carcinoma: the unusual variants. *Journal of Thoracic and Cardiovascular Surgery*, 1994; **108:** 1138.

Related topics of interest

ESOPHAGEAL CANCER: MULTIMODALITY THERAPY

Renee Kennedy, Alan G. Casson

Recent strategies to improve overall survival of patients with esophageal cancer have utilized various combinations of radiotherapy, chemotherapy and surgery. While loco-regional disease may be controlled effectively by surgery or radiotherapy, most patients eventually die of systemic (metastatic) disease, and therefore chemotherapy has assumed increasing importance in recent clinical trials.

Radiotherapy

1. Preoperative. Theoretically preoperative radotherapy can improve resection rates and sterilize the surgical field, potentially reducing loco-regional recurrence. Various preoperative radiation doses and fractions have been evaluated, predominantly for esophageal squamous cell carcinomas. Overall response rates range from 50 to 70%, with pathologic complete response in up to 20% of patients. However, disease-free and overall survival are not significantly improved with this approach. There is also no convincing evidence that preoperative radiotherapy improves resectability of esophageal tumors.

2. Postoperative. Two prospective, randomized, controlled studies have evaluated postoperative radiotherapy (55 Gy in 25 fractions; 50 Gy in 14 fractions). As no survival advantage (overall or disease-free) was seen in either study, routine postoperative radiotherapy cannot be recommended after surgical resection.

3. Brachytherapy. This technique is currently under evaluation in a variety of clinical settings, but particularly to palliate endoesophageal relapse after definitive therapy. Its role in multimodality therapy remains to be defined.

Chemotherapy

1. Single agent and combination chemotherapy. Active single agents (>20% overall response rates) in esophageal cancer (predominantly squamous cell) are: cisplatin, 5-fluorouracil, mitomycin, ifosfamide, methotrexate and bleomycin. Newer agents include paclitaxel, gemcitabine and vinorelbine. The combination of cisplatin and 5-fluorouracil has become a standard for use in esophageal cancer therapy, with reported response rates of 50% for localized disease, and 30% for metastatic disease. Combination chemotherapy may significantly improve quality of life in responders.

2. Preoperative. Induction (neo-adjuvant) chemotherapy can potentially eliminate systemic (micro-) metastases, improve resectability and evaluate tumor chemosensitivity for measurable disease. This approach is supported by studies in animal models and in several pilot clinical (Phase I/II) studies. The value of preoperative chemotherapy has not yet been determined in large, prospective, randomized clinical trials. Interim analysis of a recently completed, North American Phase III trial comparing induction chemotherapy (cisplatin, 5-fluorouracil) and surgery with surgery alone, shows no early survival advantage for either group. A comparable multicenter trial in the UK, with larger patient numbers, has recently been completed.

3. Postoperative. Few trials of postoperative (adjuvant) chemotherapy have been reported for esophageal cancer, and this approach cannot be recommended for routine clinical use.

Chemoradiotherapy

Several Phase I/II clinical trials have evaluated the efficacy of preoperative (induction) chemoradiotherapy for esophageal cancer, to enhance local and systemic disease control. Various regimens are reported, using standard chemotherapeutic agents with concurrent radiotherapy (up to 45 Gy). Studies have confirmed the feasibility of this approach, with variable results. In general, pathologic complete response rates of 20–30% are reported, with median survivals of 18–24 months. However, operative mortality rates are approximately 10%. One recent prospective, randomized, controlled clinical trial, evaluating induction chemoradiotherapy (cisplatin, 5-fluorouracil, vinblastine; 45 Gy) and surgery versus surgery alone, did not report any survival benefit. However, a much larger Phase III trial is required to evaluate this approach.

Further reading

Ajani JA. Current status of new drugs and multidisclipinary approaches in patients with carcinoma of the esophagus. *Chest*, 1998; **113 (Suppl.):** 112S.

Bosset JF, Grignoux M, Triboulet JP, Tiret E, Mantion G, Elias D, Lozarch P, Ollier JC, Pavy JJ, Mercier M, Shamoud T. Chemoradiotherapy followed by surgery compared with surgery alone in squamous-cell cancer of the esophagus. *New England Journal of Medicine*, 1997; **337:** 161.

Kelsen DP. The role of chemotherapy in the treatment of esophageal cancer. *Chest Surgery Clinics of North America*, 1994; **4:** 173.

Reed CE. Adjuvant therapy of esophageal cancer. *Annals of Thoracic Surgery*, 1997; **64:** 280.

Ruol A. Multimodality treatment for non-metastatic cancer of the thoracic esophagus. *Diseases of the Esophagus*, 1996; **9 (Suppl. 1):** 39.

Walsh TN, Noonan N, Hollywood D, Kelly A, Keeling N, Hennessy TPJ. A comparison of multimodal therapy and surgery for esophageal adenocarcinoma. *New England Journal of Medicine*, 1996; **335:** 462.

Related topics of interest

Esophageal cancer: diagnosis and staging (p. 83)

Esophageal cancer: surgery (p. 97)

ESOPHAGEAL CANCER: PALLIATION

Renee Kennedy, Alan G. Casson

The majority (50–75%) of patients with esophageal cancer will have advanced tumor stage at diagnosis, and will therefore not be suitable for curative therapy. In addition, many patients will present with significant associated general medical disease, including dehydration, malnutrition and chronic pulmonary sepsis. As survival of patients with advanced stage disease is measured in weeks to months, palliation of symptoms and maintenance of quality of life, are of utmost importance.

General

The general aims of palliation are the correction of dehydration, anemia, etc. As one aim is to restore swallowing, the use of feeding tubes (i.e. gastrostomy, jejunostomy, nasogastric) alone is of questionable value. These may be used in selected patients receiving other palliative therapies (i.e. radiotherapy) to restore swallowing. Analgesics and other pharmacologic agents are used to relieve pain, and, vigorous pulmonary therapy and appropriate antibiotics are given to treat lung infections related to chronic aspiration.

Esophageal dilation

- Commonly used, but is only of temporary value.
- Currently combined with other modes of therapy.
- See 'Esophagoscopy, dilation and stenting', p. 113.

Esophageal stents

These are used in 25–35% of all patients who present with unresectable esophageal cancer, or with malignant esophageal fistulae. Newer systems (i.e. covered self-expanding wire stents) are increasingly used with minimum morbidity and mortality, with durable long-term palliation of dysphagia. (See 'Esophagoscopy, dilation and stenting', p. 113.)

Radiation therapy

The use of external beam radiotherapy alone, for palliation of esophageal cancer, has been disappointing. Current palliative strategies, combining external beam radiotherapy with sensitizing chemotherapy (and including nutritional support, dilation or stenting), report improved swallowing in 60–80% of patients. Tumor regrowth, stricture formation and the development of malignant esophagotracheal or -bronchial fistulae are potential local failures of this approach. Early results using endoluminal brachytherapy (alone or combined with external beam) appear promising, but the precise role of this modality has not yet been defined.

Chemotherapy

Cisplatin-containing regimens produce complete or partial responses in 50–70% of patients, and may be of considerable palliative benefit. However, the duration of response varies considerably, and therefore chemotherapy is combined with other therapies (especially radiotherapy).

Laser and photodynamic therapy	Laser therapy is used as a temporary measure to restore swallowing, and should not be considered definitive local therapy. The role of photodynamic therapy is currently under evaluation.
Surgery	*1. Resection.* Surgical resection, with reconstruction of the upper gastrointestinal tract, continues to provide palliation for selected good risk patients where the perioperative mortality and morbidity are low. The decision to perform a palliative resection is generally only made at the time of surgery, when exploration reveals technically unresectable disease (primary tumor, or lymph node metastases or liver metastases).
	2. Bypass. Initial attempts at surgical bypass alone for esophageal cancers were of questionable palliative benefit. In highly selected, good-performance patients, without apparent distant metastases, with locally advanced tumors (particularly involving the respiratory tract), this option may be appropiate. Bypass is usually accomplished with the stomach placed substernally, and by excluding the esophagus and tumor. However, mortality rates are generally high (15–20%).
	3. Diversion. Proximal esophageal diversion (cervical esophagostomy, spit fistula) and feeding gastrostomy are generally considered to give poor palliation. However, this may be a reasonable approach as an initial life-saving procedure in obstructed patients with an acute esophageal perforation (usually iatrogenic).

Further reading

Dittler HJ, Pfister KGM. Stents and tubes. *Diseases of the Esophagus*, 1996; **9:** 105.

Horvath OP, Lukacs L. Palliative resection and bypass surgery. *Diseases of the Esophagus*, 1996; **9:** 117.

Minsky BD. Palliative external beam radiation therapy and combined modality therapy. *Diseases of the Esophagus*, 1996; **9:** 86.

O'Rourke IC, McNeil RJ, Walker PJ. Objective evaluation of the quality of palliation in patients with esophageal cancer comparing surgery, radiotherapy and intubation. *Australian and New Zealand Journal of Surgery*, 1992; **62:** 922.

Sawant A, Moghissi K. Management of unresectable esophageal cancer: a review of 537 patients. *European Journal of Cardiothoracic Surgery*, 1994; **8:** 113.

Spinelli P, Dal Fante M, Mancini A, Cerrai FG. Endoscopic laser therapy. *Diseases of the Esophagus*, 1996; **9:** 98.

Related topics of interest

ESOPHAGEAL CANCER: SURGERY

Renee Kennedy, Alan G. Casson

Despite poor long-term survival for esophageal cancer, surgery continues to have a prominent role in the management of this disease. Surgical resection rates vary widely, but overall, approximately 50% of patients will be judged, by preoperative staging, to have resectable disease. For early stage tumors (Tis, Stage I), complete surgical resection may be curative, with 5-year survival rates approaching 70%. For the majority of patients with locally advanced tumors, overall survival remains poor (<20% at 5 years), although considerable palliative benefit may be achieved. In recent years, surgical mortality has declined substantially and is routinely now below 5% at centers where esophagectomy is performed frequently.

Esophageal cancer diagnosis and staging

- See 'Esophageal cancer: diagnosis and staging', p. 83.
- Patients with metastatic disease (M1), or judged to have locally advanced (T4) primary tumors, are generally excluded from surgery.

Preoperative preparation

- See 'Preoperative assessment for thoracic surgery', p. 212.
- Obvious dehydration and anemia should be corrected prior to surgery.
- The value of preoperative correction of nutritional deficits is controversial, but short-term (<2 weeks) nutritional therapy does not appear to be of benefit,
- Long-term (>2 weeks) nutritional support preoperatively may correct nutritional deficiencies, but places patients at increased risk of aspiration and sepsis.

Surgical approaches

A number of approaches are described to resect esophageal cancer, varying in type and number of incisions, extent of resection, method of reconstruction and technique of anastomosis. Near-total esophagectomy (i.e. resecting the abdominal and intrathoracic esophagus) is currently preferred, for functional and oncologic reasons. The proximal extent of resection (>10 cm) should encompass submucosal tumor extension and mucosal skip lesions, requiring an anastomosis in the neck or upper chest. The extent of distal resection (especially for lower third adenocarcinomas) should be at least 5 cm, and may be guided by intraoperative frozen-section examination. To obtain clear lateral margins, a wide *en bloc* resection is preferred. This is technically more difficult to achieve using a transhiatal approach, although results are generally comparable regardless of the approach used. Extended *en bloc* resections, encompassing regional lymph-node fields, are associated with increased perioperative morbidity and moratlity, with no or minor increase in survival.

In general, surgical mortality following esophageal resection should be below 5%, regardless of the technique used.

However, the procedure has significant associated morbidity (20–40%). Commonly used approaches are summarized below.

1. Right thoracotomy/laparotomy. Laparotomy is performed initially to exclude abdominal metastasis and to mobilize the stomach. The esophagus is resected using a right thoracotomy and the correctly orientated stomach delivered through the hiatus. A high intrathoracic anastomosis is performed. If necessary, a right neck incision can be made and the gastric anastomosis made to the cervical esophagus.

2. Right thoracotomy/laparotomy/left neck. This technique is a further modification of the one given above, designed to resect the entire intrathoracic esophagus. The right thoracotomy may be performed initially to assess resectability and mobilize the tumor and esophagus along its entire length. The incision is closed and the patient positioned supine for laparotomy. The mobilized esophagus is divided and delivered through the hiatus. The stomach is then mobilized and delivered up to the left neck incision for anastomosis. Alternatively, the laparotomy and left neck incision can be performed first, and the mobilized stomach delivered substernally. The patient is repositioned for a right thoracotomy, and the esophagus and tumor are resected.

3. Left thoracotomy/thoracoabdominal. In general, left-sided approaches are used for tumors in the distal esophagus or at the esophago-gastric junction. Resection and reconstruction may be satisfactorily achieved using a left thoracotomy (incising diaphragm) or by extending the incision across the costal margin into the abdomen. Anastomosis is most frequently performed in the chest, although a left neck incision may also be utilized.

There appears to be little difference in operative mortality, morbidity and outcome, compared with right-sided approaches. Left thoracoabdominal approaches are ideal for extended gastrectomy (esophagogastrectomy) to resect proximal (i.e. fundus, cardia) gastric tumors. Reconstruction is achieved using jejunum in a Roux-en-Y configuration and an intrathoracic esophagojejunal anastomosis below the aortic arch.

4. Transhiatal (non-thoracotomy). This technique comprises resection of the intrathoracic esophagus through the esophageal hiatus (laparotomy) and the thoracic inlet (left neck), without the need for thoracotomy. The esophagus is dissected under direct vision for most of its length, although mobilization of the mid-esophagus (in the region of the carina) may be difficult. This approach is best suited for tumors of the lower esophagus (i.e. below the carina) and for gastric transposition following excision of cervical/upper esophageal cancers. One potential disadvantage of this approach relates to the extent of resection (i.e. lateral margins, *en bloc* lymphadenectomy), although survival rates are comparable with more extensive procedures.

This approach is safe when performed by an experienced surgeon. The most important intraoperative complications (<1%) are injury to the tracheobronchial tree (advance the uncut endotracheal tube beyond the injury, convert to a thoracotomy, direct repair buttressed with adjacent healthy tissues), bleeding from branches of the aorta (thoracotomy and suture) and hypotension during transhiatal mobilization (remove hand, ensure intravascular volume is adequate).

5. *VATS.* Minimally invasive approaches (i.e. thoracoscopy, laparoscopy) are increasingly used to stage esophageal cancers. Although a limited number of esophageal resections (with reconstruction) has been reported, this has not gained widespread acceptance in current practice. The most reasonable strategy described is to utilize a right-sided VATS approach to mobilize the tumor and entire intrathoracic esophagus, avoiding a formal thoracotomy. Esophageal reconstruction is achieved in the usual manner utilizing laparotomy and left neck incisions.

Esophageal reconstruction

Esophageal reconstruction should be performed at the same time as esophageal resection. The conduit of choice is the stomach, which appears to function better as a narrow tube. This is most frequently positioned in the posterior mediastinum, with an anastomosis in the left neck or upper chest. A pyloromyotomy is often performed to improve gastric drainage, but this has recently been questioned. For further details see 'Esophageal reconstruction', p. 110.

Postoperative management and complications

Careful attention to detail throughout the postoperative period is essential. It is important to anticipate potential complications, which should be diagnosed and treated early, to minimize postoperative morbidity and mortality. Routine placement of a nasogastric tube, a feeding jejunostomy, bilateral chest tubes or use of mini-tracheostomy are advocated by some surgeons. Leakage at the esophagogastric anastomosis is reported in up to 15% of cases. Intrathoracic leaks are associated with considerable morbidity and mortality, and should be treated aggressively by widespread drainage, antibiotics and nutritional support. Operative intervention to close the leak, defunction or resect the interposed conduit may be necessary. By contrast, most cervical leaks respond to local drainage. Necrosis of the gastric tip is uncommon, but will require takedown of the interposed stomach, creation of a cervical esophagostomy (spit fistula), and later reconstruction.

Other specific postoperative complications include esophageal stricture, laryngeal nerve injury injury, chylothorax, delayed mediastinal bleeding, pleural effusions and cardiac dysrhythmias. For further details see 'Postoperative management and complications', p. 206.

Further reading

Muller JM, Erasmi H, Stelzner M, Zieren U, Pilchlmaier H. Surgical therapy for esophageal carcinoma. *British Journal of Surgery*, 1990; **77**: 845.

Orringer MB, Marshall B, Sterling MC. Transhiatal esophagectomy for benign and malignant disease. *Journal of Thoracic and Cardiovascular Surgery*, 1993; **105**: 265.

Putnam JB, Suell DM, McMurtry MJ, Ryan MB, Walsh GL, Natarajan G, Roth JA. Comparison of three techniques of esophagectomy within a residency training program. *Annals of Thoracic Surgery*, 1994; **57**: 319.

Steup WH, De Leyn P, Deneffe G, Van Ramdonck D, Coosemans W, Lerut T. Tumors of the esophagogastric junction: long-term survival in relation to pattern of lymph node metastasis and a critical analysis of the accuracy of the pTNM classification. *Journal of Thoracic and Cardiovascular Surgery*, 1996; **111**: 85.

Turnbull A, Ginsberg RJ. Options in the surgical approach for esophageal carcinoma. *Chest Surgery Clinics of North America*, 1994; **57**: 315.

Related topics of interest

ESOPHAGEAL DIVERTICULA

Donna E. Maziak, F. Griff Pearson

Both true diverticula, containing all the layers of the esophageal wall, and false diverticula, containing mucosa only, can occur at any level along the esophagus. False (pulsion) diverticula are usually an anatomic manifestation (i.e. the end-result) of esophageal dysfunction, whereas true diverticula are secondary to an inflammatory process (traction).

Pharyngoesophageal (Zenker's) diverticulum

This is an acquired pulsion diverticulum, arising from a triangular weakening (Killian's triangle) in the posterior midline of the lower pharynx, between the oblique and transverse (cricopharyngeus) muscle fibers of the inferior pharyngeal constrictor. It is believed to arise as a result of cricopharyngeal (or upper esophageal) dysfunction, and the natural history is that of progressive enlargement. Patients present with dysphagia, regurgitation of undigested material and chronic aspiration, and a neck mass may be identified on examination. Diagnosis is performed by contrast studies and a careful endoscopy. Motility studies of the upper esophageal sphincter are technically difficult to perform and the results are inconsistent. Further esophageal function studies are indicated to exclude associated foregut motor disorders. Associated gastroesophageal reflux (10% patients) should be diagnosed and treated preoperatively. Surgery is curative and a left neck approach is usual. A crichophargeal myotomy is essential, dividing cricopharyngeus and extending the myotomy at least 2–3 cm onto the proximal esophagus. The extent of the upper esophageal myotomy is controversial. Larger diverticula are excised and closed transversely, with a bougie in the esophagus either by standard suture techniques or, more conveniently using a mechanical stapler. If left unexcised, suspension of the apex of the diverticulum (diverticulopexy) to the prevertebral fascia or pharyngeal musculature is advocated by some surgeons. Endoscopic treatment of the diverticulum is controversial and involves division of the septum between the posterior esophagus and the diverticulum.

Midesophageal diverticulum

Most midesophageal diverticula are traction type, secondary to mediastinal inflammatory diseases (usually granulomatous disease, i.e. tuberculosis, histoplasmosis of the subcarinal nodes). They may be associated with active inflammation, acquired tracheoesophageal fistulae and epithelialized sinus tracts. This type of diverticulum is usually asymptomatic in the absence of complications such as fistula, bleeding or abscess formation. Treatment is rarely indicated other than to manage any associated complications. This involves excision of the diverticulum, and closure of the esophagus and any associated fistula. Excision of an associated inflammatory mass may not be technically possible.

Epiphrenic diverticulum   This type of diverticulum is rare, occurring predominantly in the elderly. It is an acquired, pulsion-type, comprising a mucosal pouch protruding through the muscular wall of the lower 10 cm of the esophagus. It is most often associated with distal esophageal motility disorders (i.e. achalasia or diffuse spasm) and/or gastroesophageal reflux. Clinical presentation is variable, and no correlation exists between the severity of symptoms (i.e. dysphagia, regurgitation, chest pain, aspiration) and size of the diverticulum. Treatment is controversial – if asymptomatitc, or symptoms are minimal, no further treatment is necessary, as progression is unlikely. Surgical treatment is advised for symptomatic patients, and comprises esophageal myotomy below the diverticulum (to correct the underlying motor disorder), with excision of the divericulum. The addition of an anti-reflux procedure is controversial.

Further reading

Altorki N, Sunagawa M, Skinner DB. Thoracic esophageal diverticula: why is operation necessary? *Journal of Thoracic and Cardiovascular Surgery*, 1993; **105:** 260.

Benacci JC, Deschamps C, Trastek VF, Allen MS, Daly RC, Pairolero PC. Epiphrenic diverticulum: results of surgical treatment. *Annals of Thoracic Surgery*, 1993; **55:** 1109.

Fekete F, Vonns C. Surgical management of esophageal thoracic diverticula. *Hepatogastroenterology*, 1992; **39:** 97.

Ferguson MK. Evolution of therapy for pharyngoesophageal (Zenker's) diverticulum. *Annals of Thoracic Surgery*, 1991; **51:** 848.

Mathieu HF, deBree R, Dagli SA, Snel AM. Endoscopic treatment of Zenker's diverticulum. *Diseases of the Esophagus*, 1996; **9:** 12.

Related topics of interest

ESOPHAGEAL FUNCTION STUDIES

Donna E. Maziak, F. Griff Pearson

Objective evaluation of esophageal function is essential to define as precisely as possible the underlying pathophysiology of the foregut disorder. Esophageal symptoms may not have an anatomic basis, or may be nonspecific or atypical. Many esophageal function studies are described, but many are relatively complex and unphysiologic, and not applicable to modern practice. Recent advances in technology (miniaturized pH electrodes, pressure transducers, portable digital datarecorders) have permitted the development of ambulatory equipment to monitor the foregut over a 24-hour period in the patient's natural environment, providing further insight into esophagogastric physiology. Because of the inherent variability of these techniques and the technicians who administer the tests, it is important that each laboratory standardize techniques and define its normal values from normal volunteers.

Esophageal manometry

1. Indications
- To evaluate motility of the esophageal body.
- To evaluate function of lower esophageal sphincter (LES).
- To evaluate the pharyngoesophageal phase of swallowing (i.e. the upper esophageal sphincter, UES).

2. Technique. Esophageal manometry is performed using electronic pressure-sensitive transducers or water-perfused catheters with lateral side holes, connected to external transducers. After an overnight fast, the catheter is passed through the nose and esophagus into the stomach and the gastric pressure pattern is confirmed. The catheter is then pulled back at 0.5–1.0 cm intervals and manometric tracings are made along the entire length of the esophagus. Response to 10 wet (5 ml water) and dry swallows is also recorded.

3. Results
- LES. The respiratory inversion point is identified when the positive abdominal excursions that occur with breathing change to negative deflections in the thorax. This serves as a reference point at which the amplitude of LES pressure and the length of the sphincter exposed to abdominal pressure are measured. The pressure (median normal value, 13 mmHg), overall length (median, 3.5 cm) and length of the abdominal segment (median, 2.0 cm) are calculated. Relaxation of the LES with swallowing should also be seen. Recent developments include three-dimensional reconstruction of the LES pressure, and calculation of sphincter pressure vector volume to assess LES resistance.
- Esophageal body. Manometry is used to assess the propulsive force of the esophageal body, during dry and wet swallows. The minimum amplitude of contractions required for esophageal transit of a solid bolus range from 20 mmHg

(proximal esophagus) to 40 mmHg (lower segment). Contraction waves are classified by amplitude, duration and morphology at different levels of the esophageal body. The delay between the peak of contractions is used to calculate the speed of wave progression.

- UES. Manometric evaluation of the UES is technically difficult because of the speed of events during swallowing, asymmetry of the UES and movement of the pharynx on swallowing. Electronic pressure-sensitive transducers are preferred as they have a higher frequency response than water-perfused catheters. Specially designed catheters are now available to study UES function. Conventional studies may demonstrate insufficient relaxation or premature contractions of the UES, high UES pressures or inadequate pharyngeal pressure.

4. *Examples of abnormal patterns*
- Esophogastic junction (EGJ), i.e. achalasia. Failure of the LES to relax completely with swallowing, and the subsequent loss of progressive peristalsis in the body of the esophagus, is characteristic. A hypertensive LES is seen in about half of all patients studied. An end-stage esophagus is characterized by aperistalsis. A variant of classic achalasia (vigorous achalasia) is characterized by high-amplitude, nonperistaltic contractions. (See 'Achalasia', p. 1.)
- Esophageal body, i.e. diffuse esophageal spasm. These are frequent simultaneous and repetitive esophageal contractions, which may be of high amplitude or long duration. The esophagus retains some degree of peristaltic activity. (See 'Esophageal motor disorders', p. 107.)

5. *Ambulatory 24-hour motility.* This technique was developed to detect intermittent esophageal motor disorders, that may not be apparent during standard esophageal manometry. The primary clinical application is for the evaluation of non-cardiac chest pain. The technique is used increasingly to evaluate a spectrum of esophageal motor disorders and patients with gastroesophageal reflux disease.

Ambulatory 24-hour pH monitoring

1. *Indications*
- To detect and quantitate exposure of the lower esophagus to gastric acid.
- To test the relationship between symptoms and esophageal exposure to acidic refluxate.

2. *Technique.* A small pH electrode is passed transnasally and placed 5 cm above the upper border of the manometri-

cally defined LES. The electrode is connected to an external portable datalogger and pH values of the distal esophagus are continuously recorded at 4-s intervals for 24 hours. The patient is able to indicate the development of symptoms and times of meals. The pH in the upper esophagus may also be recorded, to obtain evidence for regurgitation into the upper esophagus and aspiration.

3. Results. Exposure of the esophageal mucosa to acidic gastric juice is assessed by the following measurements (median normal values, from 50 asymptomatic controls, are included).

- Cumulative time the esophageal pH is below a chosen threshold (usually pH 4) (1.2%). May be further analyzed by time spent upright or supine.
- Frequency of reflux episodes (16/day).
- Number of episodes greater than 5 min (0).
- Time in minutes of the longest episode (4 min).
- A composite score (DeMeester) is then calculated (based on 95th percentile at pH <4) and assigned to the patient. A value >14.7 is considered positive.

Ambulatory 24-hour bile reflux monitoring

Increasing clinical and experimental evidence has implicated the reflux of bile (or a mixed acid/bile refluxate) with esophageal mucosal injury (i.e. esophagitis), the development of Barrett's esophagus and esophageal malignancy. Existing techniques to evaluate the reflux of duodenal contents into the stomach or esophagus have been unsatisfactory. Alkaline reflux measured by pH monitoring is insensitive, as other factors may alter pH. Recently an ambulatory system (Bilitec), comprising a fiberoptic sensor probe to detect bilirubin based on its spectrophotometric properties (characteristic light absorption at 453 nm) connected to a datalogger, has been developed. This system will likely see increasing clinical application to allow precise identification of patients with bile or mixed acid/bile reflux.

Provocative tests

Applicable to only a small percentage of patients in modern clinical practice. Most have low sensitivity and specificity, and have generally been replaced by ambulatory 24-hour pH monitoring.

1. Acid perfusion test (Berstein test). Indicated to determine whether symptoms are reproduced by the infusion of acid into the esophagus. The distal esophagus is perfused with 0.1 N HCl at 6–8 ml/min, alternating with a placebo (i.e. saline). The patient is asked to report any symptom that develops during the infusion. A positive test is consistent reproduction of symptoms only during acid perfusion, with rapid alleviation during saline perfusion or after administration of an antacid.

2. *Edrophonium (Tensilon) test.* Developed to identify chest pain of esophageal origin, following an IV injection of edrophonium hydrochloride (a cholinesterase inhibitor).

3. *Balloon distention test.* An inflatable balloon is positioned in the lower esophagus and gradually inflated. The test is positive when typical symptoms are reproduced, confirming an esophageal origin of chest pain.

Other tests

1. *Video radiography.* To qualitatively evaluate swallowing of liquids and solids, and gastroesophageal reflux. Particularly useful to evaluate UES function.

2. *Radionuclide scintigraphy.* To semiquantitate esophageal transit, gastroesophageal reflux, gastric emptying and bile reflux. Lack of standardization has limited widespread application of many of these studies.

Further reading

Bonavina L, Evander A, DeMeester TR, Walther B, Cheng SC, Palazzo L, Concannon JL. Length of the distal esophageal sphincter and competency of the cardia. *American Journal of Surgery*, 1986; **151:** 25.

Stein HJ, DeMeester TR, Hinder RA. Outpatient physiologic testing and surgical management of foregut motility disorders. In: Wells SA, ed. *Current Problems in Surgery*. St. Louis: Mosby-Year Book, 1992; 425.

Stein HJ, DeMeester TR, Naspetti R, Jamieson J, Perry RE. Three-dimensional imaging of the lower esophageal sphincter in gastroesophageal reflux disease. *Annals of Surgery*, 1991; **214:** 374.

Related topics of interest

ESOPHAGEAL MOTOR DISORDERS

Donna E. Maziak, F. Griff Pearson

Functional disorders of the esophageal body and lower esophageal sphincter may give rise to pain, dysphagia, or interfere with normal swallowing, but are not associated with any organic obstruction of the esophagus. Esophageal motility disorders have traditionally been classified as primary or secondary. Although each disorder may have characteristic clinical, radiographic and manometric findings, there is considerable overlap between each entity. Every effort must therefore be made to establish as precise a diagnosis as possible, and to understand the pathophysiology of esophageal dysfunction. Surgical modification of foregut anatomy, to correct esophageal function, may be particularly challenging, and careful patient selection is necessary to ensure a good outcome.

Primary motor disorders

Primary motor disorders of the esophagus are characterized by abnormal esophageal motility without associated systemic disease. They may broadly be characterized by hypermotility (i.e. nutcracker esophagus, diffuse esophageal spasm) where functional obstruction, dysphagia and pain are the primary symptoms; or by hypomotility (i.e. hypotensive LES) where gastroesophageal reflux predominates. The pathophysiology of these disorders is largely unknown, but may arise as a result of abnormal esophageal muscle, or altered response to neurotransmitters or circulating hormones. At present, therapy for primary esophageal motor disorders is usually nonspecific, and includes anticholinergic agents, calcium-channel blockers, nitrates, empiric dilation and occasionally surgery.

Diffuse esophageal spasm This is a disorder characterized by abnormal esophageal motility, chest pain or dysphagia. Patients may have a characteristic barium study, showing segmentation, pseudodiverticulum or a 'corkscrew' appearance. The manometric criteria for diagnosis are controversial, but the most widely accepted definition requires the presence of an increased frequency of simultaneous (nonperistaltic) contractions in the body of the esophagus, with some preservation of the normal peristaltic function. Other manometric findings may include high-amplitude, repetitive or prolonged-duration contractions. Initial management involves the use of nitrates or calcium-channel blockers. Patients with severe symptoms not responding to medical treatment may require pneumatic dilatation or surgical myotomy. If a surgical myotomy is performed, it usually extends from the proximal extent of the esophageal smooth mucscle onto the stomach. It is controversial whether an anti-reflux procedure should be performed.

Nutcracker esophagus This is a manometrically defined syndrome characterized by high-amplitude (>180 mmHg) peristaltic contractions in the body of the esophagus. Patients present with chest pain and dysphagia. Although barium studies and esophagoscopy should be performed to rule out other esophageal disorders, manometry is required to make the diagnosis. Treatment is with calcium-channel blockers and anticholinergic agents. In general, dilation or surgery (i.e. myotomy) has not been helpful.

Hypertensive lower esophageal sphincter

This isolated dysfunction of the LES, characterized by hypertension (>45 mmHg), and poor relaxation, is recognized as a separate entity. Half of all patients will have normal peristalsis in the esophageal body, but a 'nutcracker'-like appearance may also be identified. Patients present with chest pain and dysphagia. Management should initially be pharmacologic, although selected patients may benefit from esophageal dilation (rarely surgery). All patients should be followed long-term to exclude further deterioration in esophageal function.

Nonspecific esophageal motility disorders

This is a diagnosis of exclusion in patients with complaints of dysphagia and chest pain, who do have specific manometric criteria to diagnose a primary esophageal motor disorder. Manometry is clearly abnormal, and may identify multi-peaked, repetitive, spontaneous and prolonged contractions. Secondary causes should be excluded.

Achalasia

See 'Achalasia', p. 1.

Secondary motor disorders

Gastroesophageal reflux disease (GERD)

This is the most common disorder leading to esophageal body dysfunction and it may be difficult to distinguish preoperatively from a primary motor disorder. Although GERD has a multifactorial etiology, incompetence of the LES has been reported in 60–70% of patients. Effective anti-reflux therapy (including surgery) may improve secondary esophageal motor disorders.

Associated with systemic disease

- Scleroderma (see below).
- Diabetes mellitus.
- Amyloidosis.
- Mixed connective tissue diseases.
- Polymyositis.
- Dermatomyositis.

Scleroderma. This is a chronic connective-tissue disorder, resulting in abnormal collagen deposits and fibrosis in the GI tract, particularly affecting the smooth muscle of the distal esophagus. Patients complain of dysphagia (liquids and solids), and severe reflux leading to erosive esophagitis and peptic stricture. Evaluation of this disorder is by barium swallow, esophagogastroscopy and esophageal function studies, including manometry. Typical manometric findings include normal proximal peristalsis (corresponding to striated muscle location), and weak or absent peristalsis in the distal two-thirds. The LES is hypotensive or absent, and significant gastroesophageal reflux may be documented. Treatment is directed towards GERD (antacids) and associated stricture (dilation; surgery). For patients refractory to medical therapy (particularly with stricture), anti-reflux surgery may be required.

Further reading

Duranceau A. Motor disorders of the esophagus. *Annals of Thoracic Surgery*, 1993; **55:** 1273.

Duranceau A, Pera M. Motor disorders of the esophagus. *Diseases of the Esophagus,* 1995; **8:** 159.

Henderson RD. Esophageal motor disorders. *Surgery Clinics of North America*, 1987; **67:** 455.

Walker SJ. What's new in pathology, pathophysiology and management of benign esophageal disorders? *Diseases of the Esophagus,* 1997; **10:** 282.

Related topics of interest

ESOPHAGEAL RECONSTRUCTION

Renee Kennedy, Alan G. Casson

Successful reconstruction of the upper GI tract following esophageal resection of benign and malignant disease, remains a technical challenge. The aim of surgery is to restore swallowing (and quality of life), and ideally reconstruction should be performed immediatley following resection, at the same operation. The stomach, colon and jejunum have all been used successfully to replace the esophagus, but practical considerations favor the use of stomach in the majority of situations.

Stomach

The stomach is easily mobilized by dividing the short gastric vessels, the left gastric artery and vein, while retaining an excellent blood supply, based on the right gastroepiploic artery (and to a lesser extent, the right gastric artery). Blood supply to the tip of the gastric conduit may be optimized by dissecting into the splenic hilum to preserve anastomoses between the gastroepiploic and short gastric vessels, and creating a narrow gastric tube (rather than using whole stomach). Additional length can be obtained by dividing the lateral attachments of the first and second parts of duodenum (Kocher maneuver), performing a pyloromyotomy rather than a pyloroplasty, application of the mechanical stapler to resect the lesser curve to create a narrow gastric tube (of the greater curvature), and using the most direct route (posterior mediastinum) to position the stomach. Care should be taken to ensure correct orientation of the stomach during transposition, to avoid volvulus and mechanical gastric outlet obstruction or vascular compromise. Only one anastomosis is required, which may be performed by a variety of techniques. Long-term function of the stomach is satisfactory in the majority of patients, with appropiate dietary manipulation. Reduced capacity, delayed emptying and reflux are the most common postoperative functional disorders.

Gastric tubes. Various reversed and nonreversed gastric tubes, each based on a defined blood supply, have been described. In adult practice, they appear to offer few advantages over stomach transposition and require considerably longer to create. Most have been used in pediatric surgical practice.

Colon

The colon is the most commonly used alternative to the stomach, in patients who have had previous gastric surgery, or if the stomach is involved with tumor. An isoperistaltic segment of left colon, based on the inferior mesenteric artery is preferred, and additional length may be obtained by using transverse colon (preserving anastomotic arcades with middle colic vessels and the marginal artery). Colon can not be used in the presence of intrinsic colonic disease (excluded by preoperative barium enema and colonoscopy) or with a compromised vascular supply (evaluated by angiography). A further disadvantage is greater operating time, as three anastomoses (esophagocolic; cologastric or jejunal and colocolic) are required.

Jejunum

Isoperistaltic jejunal loops (or Roux-en-Y reconstruction) have been used to replace the lower esophagus. Their main disadvantage is limited mobility, but with careful preservation of mesenteric vascular arcades, they may be mobilized (tension free) to at least the level of the hilum.

Free jejunal transfer. Free jejunal grafts have been used successfully to replace the upper esophagus (above the thoracic inlet, after hypopharyngeal resection. A precise microvascular anastomosis is generally required to obtain a successful graft.

Skin/myocutaneous flaps

Early attempts at esophageal reconstruction (predominantly in the neck) utilized various skin or myocutaneous flaps (i.e. pectoralis major myocutaneous flap). Generally poor functional results have limited their routine use. They are occasionally used to control anastomotic leaks or fistulae.

Route

1. Posterior mediastinum. Placing the interposed stomach or colon in the bed of the resected esophagus is the most direct route to the upper esophagus, and is used most frequently.

2. Retrosternal. Useful for situations where the posterior mediastinal route is not accessible (i.e. delayed reconstruction) or when postoperative radiotherapy to the esophageal bed is planned. It is important to enlarge the thoracic inlet (i.e. resect the medial clavicle, first rib and a portion of the manubrium) to prevent proximal obstruction.

3. Transpleural. Used during left thoracotomy to perform a high thoracic anastomosis lateral to the aortic arch. Otherwise, this route has limited application.

4. Subcutaneous. Used infrequently; has few obvious advantages.

Further reading

Ancona E, Pianalto S, Merigliano S, Peracchia A. Esophageal reconstruction: free jejunal transfer for the reconstruction of the pharyngo-esophagus. *Diseases of the Esophagus*, 1995; **8**: 40.

Casson AG, Powe J, Inculet RI, Finley R. Functional results of gastric interposition following total esophagectomy. *Clinical Nuclear Medicine*, 1991; **16**: 918.

Little AG. Esophageal reconstruction: location of the interposition. *Diseases of the Esophagus*, 1995; **8**: 4.

Mansour KA, Bryan FC, Carlson GW. Bowel interposition for esophageal replacement: twenty-five-year experience. *Annals of Thoracic Surgery*, 1997; **64:** 752.

McLarty AJ, Deschamps C, Trastek VF, Allen MS, Pairolero PC, Harmsen WS. Esophageal resection for cancer of the esophagus: long-term function and quality of life. *Annals of Thoracic Surgery*, 1997; **63:** 1568.

Siewert JR, Stein HJ, Liebermann-Meffert D, Bartels H. Esophageal reconstruction: the gastric tube as esophageal substitute. *Diseases of the Esophagus* 1995; **8:** 11.

Thomas P, Fuentes P, Giudicelli R, Reboud E. Colon interposition for esophageal replacement: current indications and long-term function. *Annals of Thoracic Surgery*, 1997; **64:** 757.

Related topics of interest

ESOPHAGOSCOPY, DILATION AND STENTING

Shaf Keshafjee, Hani K. Najm

Esophagoscopy, dilation and stenting are commonly performed procedures, for the diagnosis and treatment of a diverse spectrum of esophageal disorders. It is recommended that a radiologic contrast study is performed prior to esophageal instrumentation, to define foregut anatomy, especially distal to a narrow stricture. Although these techniques appear quite straightforward, considerable experience is required to perform these procedures with safety.

Esophagoscopy

Fiberoptic esophagoscopy Use of a flexible fiberoptic esophagogastroscope may be performed using local anesthesia on a conscious (or sedated) patient, with minimal discomfort. It may also be performed under general anesthesia. This technique allows excellent visualization of the foregut, from cricopharyngeus to the second part of the duodenum. Retroflexion of the scope is essential to examine the gastric fundus and the esophagogastric junction. Recent advances in imaging permit photography, and biopsies, brush cytology, endoscopic electrocoagulation, laser, cutting or grasping objects may all be performed readily using this technique. Dilatation of a stricture, using a balloon or over a guidewire (with or without the aid of fluroscopy) may also be performed.

Rigid esophagoscopy
- Usually requires a general anesthetic.
- Visualization is limited to the esophagus only.
- Larger biopsies may be obtained.
- Useful for therapeutic applications: facilitates safe removal of foreign bodies, allows efficient clearance of blood with large suction tubes, and for direct esophageal dilation.

Diagnostic applications
- To evaluate the esophageal mucosa for evidence of esophagitis.
- To stage the degree of mucosal injury following ingestion of a corrosive substance.
- For evidence of Barrett's epithelium.
- Biopsy any mucosal abnormalities, benign or malignant.
- Brushing of any abnormal area for screening for early detection of esophageal cancer in high-risk patients.
- Investigation of intrathoracic congenital malformations.
- Staging of esophageal malignancy.
- To evaluate an esophageal anastomosis.
- To evaluate response to therapy (i.e. healing of an ulcer).

Therapeutic applications Therapeutic applications of esophagoscopy include: removal of foreign bodies; the insertion of a feeding tube into the esophagus or stomach (percutaneous gastrostomy) under direct vision; placement of a brachytherapy catheter; and sclerotherapy of esophageal or gastric varices.

The technique can also be used for hemostatis following an endoscopic procedure (i.e. biopsy, polypectomy, sclerotherapy) or spontaneous bleeding (i.e. varices, ulcers, malignant tumors). This may be performed with a local injection with normal saline, epinephrine (1:10 000 dilution) or a sclerosing agent (1% ethoxysclerol); application of a neodymium–yttrium aluminium garnet (Nd-YAG) laser to the bleeding point; or insertion a balloon catheter for tamponade.

Further uses include resection of small esophageal mucosal and submucosal tumors, such as papillomas, granulomatous polyps, fibromas, lipomas, granular cell tumors or cysts; the, dilation of esophageal strictures; the insertion of esophageal stents; and facilitation of photodynamic therapy for early carcinomas of the esophagus (*in situ* and microinvasive squamous cell carinomas) in selected patients.

Esophageal dilation

Dilators

- *Balloon.* Produces a radial force evenly applied along the stricture.
- *Bougie.* A semirigid, flexible and tapered instrument, which applies a radial and lingitudinal force. Several types are available: nonguided (i.e. gum-elastic tipped Jackson bougies; tapered Maloney dilators) or guided (i.e. Savary–Galliard).

Technique

The aim of dilation is to increase the diameter of the esophageal lumen. The choice of dilator depends on the stricture, operator preference and availability. This technique may be performed under general or local anesthesia. Gradual dilation is essential and considerable judgement is required. It is better to redilate a stricture 1 week later than to risk excessive dilation (and perforation) at the first attempt. A rule of thumb is that dilation should cease once blood is noted on the dilator. Patients should be monitored during recovery. Any suspicion of perforation warrants further investigation (i.e. contrast study).

Complications

- Esophageal perforation. An uncommon complication, which may occur despite meticulous technique.
- Bleeding.
- Distant sepsis (i.e. bacteremia, cerebral abscess, endocarditis, septic arthritis).

Esophageal stenting

Stents

A variety of endoluminal prostheses are available to stent obstructing esophageal tumors, or to occlude malignant esophagorespiratory fistulae. Effective palliation of dysphagia using esophageal stenting is achieved in at least two-thirds of patients, although median survival of patients is about 4 months. Semirigid plastic tubes (i.e. Wilson–Cook, Atkinson) may be placed endoscopically, and selected individually, based on the length of the tumor and the degree of obstruction. Self-expanding wire stents (i.e. Gianturco) may be placed endoscopically or under radiologic control, with a resulting esophageal lumen of up to 20 mm. Newer covered stents prevent tumor ingrowth and are compatible with radiotherapy.

Techniques

The pulsion (or push) technique is commonly used, under local or general anesthesia. A barium contrast study and esophagoscopy are required to assess the extent of the primary tumor. Dilation is performed over a guidewire (Savary technique) to 2 F larger than the stent. The stent is mounted on an introducer and carefully advanced using a plastic rod across the tumor. Stents should be placed 2–3 cm longer than the proximal and distal margins of the tumor. The procedure may be performed under fluoroscopy and the position of the stent should be confirmed endoscopically. Stents may be placed at laparotomy using a traction (or pull) technique through a gastrotomy. Self-expanding stents require minimal tumor dilation, and are placed using the manufacturer's delivery system.

Complications

Postoperative mortality rates, usually due to perforation, are around 8%, and approximately 10% of patients will experience stent-related difficulties including obstruction by a food bolus, stent migration, esophageal fistulae (arising from pressure necrosis) and gastroesophageal reflux. Mortality and morbidity may be reduced with self-expanding covered stents, with a durable palliation of dysphagia.

Further reading

Feins RH, ed. Thoracic endoscopy. *Chest Surgery Clinics of North America*, 1996; **6**: 161.

Good S, Asch MR, Jaffer N, Casson AG. Radiologic placement of metallic esophageal stents: preliminary experience. *Canadian Association of Radiology Journal* 1997; **48**: 340.

Savary M, Monnier P. Esophagoscopy. In: Pearson FG, Deslauriers J, Ginsberg RJ, Hiebert CA, McKneally MF, Urschel HC, eds. *Esophageal Surgery*. New York: Churchill Livingstone, 1995; 105.

Related topics of interest

EXTENDED PULMONARY RESECTION

Sean Grondin, Michael R. Johnston

Lung cancer can be locally aggressive and invade adjacent intrathoracic structures. To provide potentially curative surgical therapy the surgeon may have to extend the limits of conventional pulmonary resection, with an *en bloc* excision of contiguous intrathoracic structures. The best long-term results are achieved in the absence of lymph node metastases, and following a complete excision, with clear histologic margins around the tumor. Common intrathoracic structures invaded by lung cancer are discussed below.

Chest wall

Chest-wall invasion designates a tumor as T3, which does not preclude resection. *En bloc* resection of lung and chest wall results in 5-year survival rates of 30–40% if mediastinal nodes (N2) are not involved. Reconstruction with prosthetic material may be necesssary. Postoperative radiotherapy is advocated by some oncologists to decrease the local recurrence rate but controlled clinical trials supporting this treatment are lacking.

Pericardium

Tumors within the lung hilum can invade directly into the pericardium, and the pulmonary artery, pulmonary veins and phrenic nerve may also be involved. In such cases, wide excision of the pericardium and involved structures is often feasible. Primary closure or reconstruction of the pericardium with synthetic patch material is recommended to prevent cardiac herniation.

Diaphragm

Diffuse diaphragmatic involvement precludes resection. Direct invasion of the diaphragm from lung cancer can be included in an *en bloc* resection of the primary tumor with acceptable results. Small defects are closed primarily, whereas larger defects require reconstruction with prosthetic material to prevent abdominal organ herniation into the chest.

Vertebral body

Direct tumor invasion of the vertebral body may cause back pain or neurologic symptoms. Involvement of the body usually precludes curative resection, although this may be technically possible using an osteotome. Transverse processes may be resected *en bloc* relatively easily to obtain a complete local excision. However, palliative radiotherapy is the treatment of choice.

Superior vena cava (SVC)

Tumor invasion may present with SVC obstruction, and such invasion usually signifies advanced nodal disease and precludes resection. When a primary lung tumor (usually the anterior segment of the right upper lobe) invades the SVC, resection of the vein may be carried out with long-term survival, if the mediastinal lymph nodes are not involved. A ribbed PTFE graft or an autologous vein patch may be used in reconstruction of the SVC.

Esophagus

Lung cancer with direct esophageal invasion is uncommon, however, metastatic subcarinal lymph nodes (N2) may cause extrinsic compression and dysphagia, or may invade directly. Palliation of dysphagia by esophageal stent placement is helpful and is usually well tolerated. Radiation therapy (or chemoradiotherapy) may also improve symptoms but runs the risk of tracheoesophageal fistula formation.

Further reading

Darteville PG. Extended operations for the treatment of lung cancer. *Annals of Thoracic Surgery*, 1997; **63:** 12.

Luketich JD, van Raemdonch DE, Ginsberg RJ. Extended resections for higher-stage non-small cell lung cancer. *World Journal of Surgery*, 1993; **17:** 719.

McCaughan BC. Primary lung cancer invading the chest wall. *Chest Surgery Clinics of North America*, 1994; **4:** 17.

Naruke T. Bronchoplastic and bronchovascular procedures of the tracheobronchial tree in the management of primary lung cancer. *Chest*, 1989; **96 (Suppl.):** 53S.

Related topics of interest

Chest-wall reconstruction (p. 46)
Lung cancer: surgery (p. 154)
Pancoast tumors (p. 184)
Superior vena cava syndrome (p. 232)

FOREIGN BODIES OF THE AERODIGESTIVE TRACT

Shaf Keshafjee, Hani K. Najm

Foreign bodies are aspirated or swallowed most often by infants or by susceptible adults. In general, up to 25% of all foreign bodies become impacted in the airway and the remainder in the digestive tract. Of those foreign bodies in the airway, 20% impact at the glottis, 7% in the trachea, 48% in the right mainstem bronchus and 25% in the left mainstem bronchus. A history of foreign body aspiration or ingestion should be investigated even when there are no overt clinical manifestations. Failure to manage foreign bodies appropiately may lead to serious and often life-threatening complications.

Airway

Evaluation

1. History. Foreign-body aspiration may be witnessed directly (for example, by a parent) or suspected. A history of previous aspiration may be obtained. Infants and children are at high risk. However, susceptible adult populations include the mentally handicapped, epileptics and alcoholics.

2. Examination. Presentation may range from acute respiratory distress (obstruction) to normal. Respiratory tract symptoms such as a sudden onset, or unexplained, wheezing, cough or recurrent pneumonias, should be investigated further.

3. Radiology. The foreign body may be visualized on postero-anterior (PA) and lateral X-rays of the chest and neck. Occasionally CT scanning may be useful, especially if the foreign body is long-standing, and local tissue reaction, stricture or complications (i.e. migration through the wall; distal pneumonia) have developed.

4. Bronchoscopy. Flexible fiberoptic, or rigid bronchoscopy is used to confirm the presence of a foreign body, its geometry and orientation, and anatomic location within the tracheo-bronchial tree.

Management

Removal of the foreign body from the airway:

- Rigid bronchoscopy, under general anesthesia.
- A vareity of foreign-body forceps should be available.
- If the object is too large to pass through the lumen of the bronchoscope, maintain a firm grip with the forceps and withdraw the instrument, forceps and foreign body as one unit.
- A balloon catheter may be passed beyond a foreign body, inflated and pulled back to dislodge it.

- Reinsert the bronchoscope (rigid or flexible) into the airway after removal of foreign body to ensure complete removal and to exclude iatrogenic injury.

Complications
- Local inflammation, granulation and fibrosis, with airway obstruction and subsequent distal pneumonia.
- Hemoptysis.
- Tension pnuemonthorax, when the foreign body acts as a ball-valve causing hyperinflation with every breath.

Foregut

Most ingested foreign bodies pass spontaneously, although it is estimated that 10–20% will require endoscopic removal and 1% surgical removal. The following sites of anatomic narrowing are the most frequent sites of impaction.

- Cricopharyngeus.
- At the level of the aortic arch.
- At the level of the left mainstem bronchus.
- Above the esophagogastric junction.
- At any level of pathologic narrowing (i.e. tumor) or extrinsic compression (i.e. enlarged mediastinal lymph nodes).

Complications arising from ingested foreign bodies include obstruction, bleeding, ulceration, perforation and mediastinitis.

Evaluation

1. History. As for the airway, a high index of suspicion should be maintained in children and 'at risk' adults. The latter also include prison or psychiatric hospital inmates, who may deliberately ingest a variety of foreign bodies. Drug smugglers who ingest packaged drugs pose a particular risk to patient and surgeon alike.

2. Examination. Manifestations include dysphagia, odynophagia (pain on swallowing), drooling (unable to swallow saliva), bleeding, chest pain or respiratory symptoms from airway compression (uncommon).

3. Radiology. PA and lateral plain X-rays are useful. Contrast studies may be useful to confirm the presence and location of the foreign body, to image coexisting pathology (i.e. tumor) and to exclude a perforation.

4. Esophagogastroscopy. Flexible fiberoptic esophagogastroscopy is useful just prior to instrumentation with the rigid esophagoscope, to confirm the nature, site and orientation of the foreign body.

Management

Removal of the foreign body from the foregut. It is occasionally suggested that foreign bodies should be pushed into the stomach using a nasogastric tube or endoscope, in the hope they will pass spontaneously. In general this is a dangerous maneuver, as further damage and perforation may occur. The following techniques should be used.

- Rigid esophagoscopy, under general anesthesia.
- The patient is positioned head-down (Trendelenberg) to avoid lodgement in the larynx during extraction.
- Open pins (cephalad) may be cautiously advanced into the stomach, rotated, and withdrawn to avoid perforation from the sharp tip.
- Surgical removal should be considered for sharp objects and drug-filled condoms to avoid rupture.
- A contrast study (water soluble followed by dilute barium) should be performed after the procedure, if any suspicion of perforation exists.

Further reading

Kelly SM, Marsh BR. Airway foreign bodies. *Chest Surgery Clinics of North America*, 1996; **6**: 253.

Smitheringale A. Foreign bodies in the respiratory tract. In: Pearson FG, Deslauriers J, Ginsberg RJ, Hiebert CA, McKneally MF, Urschel HC, eds. *Thoracic Surgery*. New York: Churchill Livingstone, 1995; 1591.

Related topics of interest

GASTROESOPHAGEAL REFLUX DISEASE

Donna E. Maziak, F. Griff Pearson

Gastroesophageal reflux is the passage of gastric contents across the esophagogastric junction into the lower esophagus. This occurs in most normal individuals to some extent, and may be regarded as a physiologic process. Several factors (anatomic and physiologic) contribute to competence of the esophagogastric junction. Pathologic gastroesophageal reflux has a multi-factorial etiology and manifests when a patient becomes symptomatic, or develops progressive inflammatory changes in the wall of the esophagus (i.e. esophagitis). Although the natural history of gastroesophageal reflux disease (GERD) is not known, it is estimated that 46% of patients will experience one isolated episode, 31% will develop recurrent nonprogressive disease and 23% will develop recurrent progressive disease, associated with complications, including ulcerative esophagitis and stricture, aspiration, or the development of a columnar-epithelium-lined (Barrett's) esophagus.

Prevalence

- GERD accounts for approximately 75% of all esophageal disease.
- The prevalence of reflux esophagitis at endoscopy ranges from 0.5 to 25%.
- It is most prevalent in adults, predominantly in males.
- The prevalence of reflux esophagitis varies geographically, but is generally high (>20%) throughout the western world. Ethnic and socioeconomic factors may contribute.
- An increased prevalence of reflux esophagitis has been reported from several centers. However, this may reflect wider availability of upper GI endoscopy.

Etiology and pathophysiology

The pathophysiology of GERD is controversial, and likely has a multifactorial etiology. It is likely that different factors assume varying importance in individual patients. However, the most common cause of GERD (and its complications) is thought to be a mechanically defective LES.

1. Lower esophageal sphincter (LES). Several anatomic factors have been proposed to contribute to the competence of the LES. The most important appears to be the length of the intra-abdominal esophagus, although diaphragmatic compression, the acute angle (of His) between the esophagus and gastric fundus, mucosal folds and gastric sling fibers may contribute. An anatomic sphincter is not seen in humans.

There is continued controversy about the significance of an associated sliding hiatus hernia in contributing to pathologic GERD.

Incompetence of the LES is thought to be the main factor contributing to GERD; it is found in over 50% of patients with increased esophageal exposure to acid, and is associated with the development of GERD-related complications. It is thought to arise by either inappropriate LES relaxation or hypotensive LES.

- Inappropriate LES relaxation. This is thought to be the most significant factor, although the etiology is unknown. Appropiate LES relaxation occurs in response to peristalsis, and although transient LES relaxation is seen frequently in normal individuals (a physiologic reflex and mechanism of belching), the stimulus and mechanism of LES relaxation is not fully understood. Transient inappropiate LES relaxation is seen in the majority of patients with GERD, where it is thought to occur as a primary disorder.
- Hypotensive LES. Low basal LES is associated with spontaneous reflux and increasing severity of esophagitis. It is thought to occur as a primary disorder, but may result from esophageal tissue damage and inflammation.

2. Nature of the refluxate. Acid and pepsin (gastric juice) are the major contributors to esophageal mucosal damage. Reflux of the duodenal contents (bile acids and salts, usually mixed with gastric acid/pepsin) has recently been implicated in the development of esophagitis and Barrett's mucosa.

3. Esophageal mucosal resistance. The normal esophageal mucosa is able to withstand brief episodes of acid reflux which occur daily in normal individuals. The presence of bicarbonate ions in the esophageal mucus is thought to be the most important protective mechanism, although epithelial-cell-membrane permeability, intracellular buffers and local esophageal blood flow may contribute.

4. Esophageal clearance mechanisms. Loss of any of the following mechanisms can increase esophageal exposure to refluxed material.

- Gravity. This mechanism is lost while supine. While asleep, reduced salivation and decreased peristalsis may also contribute to reduced esophageal clearance.
- Peristalsis (esophageal motor activity). Refluxed material is generally cleared by secondary peristalsis, initiated by lower esophageal distention or reduced intraesophageal pH. Esophageal peristalsis is abnormal in a significant number of patients with GERD (likely a secondary event), but conversely, GERD may be severe in patients with primary esophageal motor disorders (i.e. scleroderma).
- Salivation. Alkaline saliva has a neutralizing effect on refluxed acid that is not cleared by peristalsis or gravity.
- Intra-abdominal esophagus. The presence of a sliding hiatus hernia with a shortened esophagus is associated with

inadequate esophageal clearance and prolonged esophageal transit time (abnormal hiatal flow).

5. *Abnormal gastric function.* Delayed gastric emptying is found in over 50% of patients with GERD. Gastric dilation or distention stimulates further acid secretion and reduces LES pressure, accentuating gastroesophageal reflux.

6. *Miscellaneous conditions associated with GERD*
- Pregnancy (mechanical and hormone effects).
- Previous gastric surgery.
- Zollinger–Ellison syndrome.
- Treated achalasia.
- Nasogastric intubation.
- Scleroderma.
- Diabetes mellitus.

Complications of GERD

1. *Peptic esophagitis*
- Mucosal inflammation/ulceration.
- Peptic stricture/acquired short esophagus.
- Acquired columnar epithelium-lined (Barrett's) esophagus.

2. *Motor dysfunction*
- Impared LES function.
- Impared peristalsis (esophageal body).

3. *Aspiration*
- Pharyngitis/laryngitis.
- Tracheobronchitis.
- Asthma.
- Pneumonitis/bronchiectasis/pulmonary fibrosis.

Clinical presentation

The classic symptoms of GERD are heartburn and regurgitation. However, a wide range of additional symptoms may be reported. Occasional patients, with objective evidence of significant acid reflux or esophagitis, may be asymptomatic. Symptoms of the complications of GERD include dysphagia (usually indicating a stricture, occasionally a functional disorder), cough, wheeze, loss of voice, water brash, globus, pneumonia (indicating aspiration), bleeding and anemia (ulcerative esophagitis).

Diagnosis

One single investigation can not evaluate all aspects of GERD, and therefore the following studies should be considered complementary, providing quantitation of abnormal acid (or bile) reflux, assessment of esophageal mucosal damage and the identification of associated motor disorders.

1. *Radiology.* Plain CXR is usually normal, but may occasionally show evidence of aspiration pneumonia and of an air/fluid level in the mediastinum suggestive of an associated

hiatus hernia. Contrast studies of the foregut (to evaluate functional disorders) are generally underrated. A barium swallow will demonstrate the anatomy of the esophagus and stomach, associated abnormalities (i.e. Schatzki's ring, stricture, tumor, peptic ulceration) and, depending on the technique, mucosal disease (i.e. esophagitis). Video-fluoroscopy can provide valuable information (qualitative) about swallowing and reflux.

2. Esophagoscopy. Flexible fiberoptic esophagogastroscopy is the optimal technique to assess the extent of mucosal disease. Several classifications (and modifications) are currently in use, including that proposed by Skinner and Belsey (1967).

- Stage I: mucosal redenning without ulceration.
- Stage II: linear ulceration in squamous epithelium.
- Stage III: confluent superficial erosions, becoming circumferential.
- Stage IV: peptic stricture.

A more recent classification (Armstrong *et al.*, 1991) encompasses all aspects of mucosal damage: metaplasia (M), ulcers (U), stricture (S) and erosions (E). In the MUSE classification, each category is scored to obtain objective quantitation of lesions.

Biopsy is primarily of value to exclude malignancy, and to diagnose Barrett's mucosa and evaluate dysplastic change. Histologic grading of esophagitis has been unsatisfactory.

Dilation of peptic strictures may be performed at the time of initial endoscopy.

3. Esophageal function studies. Ambulatory 24-hour pH studies are used to detect and quantitate exposure of the lower esophagus to gastric acid, and to test the relationship between reflux events and symptoms. A composite score (DeMeester) >14.7 is considered positive. Manometry is used to evaluate esophageal motor function and to evaluate the LES. An incompetent LES is characterized by a median pressure of less than 6 mmHg, an overall length of less than 2 cm, with less than 1 cm of intra-abdominal esophagus. Other studies, including ambulatory bile reflux monitoring, radionuclide esophageal transit and reflux studies may be useful in selected patients. For further information, see 'Esophageal function studies', p. 103.

Management

See 'Anti-reflux surgery', p. 12 and 'Gastroesophageal reflux disease: medical management', p. 127.

Further reading

Armstrong D, Emde C, Inauen W, Blum AL. Diagnostic assessment of gastroesophageal reflux disease: what is possible vs. what is practical? *Hepato-gastroenterology*, 1992; **39:** 3.

Armstrong D, Monnier P, Nicolet M, Blum AL, Savary M. Endoscopic assessment of esophagitis. *Gullet*, 1991; **1:** 63.

Ollyo JB, Monnier P, Fontolliet C, Savary M. The natural history, prevalence and incidence of reflux esophagitis. *Gullet*, 1993; **3:** 3.

Pope CE. Acid-reflux disorders. *New England Journal of Medicine*, 1994; **331:** 656.

Sivri B, McCallum RW. What has the surgeon to know about the pathophysiology of reflux disease? *World Journal of Surgery*, 1992; **16:** 294.

Skinner DB, Belsey R. Surgical management of esophageal reflux and hiatal hernia: long-term results with 1030 patients. *Journal of Thoracic and Cardiovascular Surgery*, 1967; **53:** 33.

Related topics of interest

GASTROESOPHAGEAL REFLUX DISEASE: MEDICAL MANAGEMENT

Donna E. Maziak, F. Griff Pearson

All patients with GERD are treated medically at some stage. For many, particularly with uncomplicated GERD, this is the only therapy required. It is important to approach the medical therapy of GERD in a logical manner to achieve maximal efficacy.

Lifestyle modification

- Elevate the head of the bed on 6-inch blocks; this allows the effect of gravity to help in esophageal clearance.
- Weight loss in obese patients; it is believed that an increase in abdominal pressure found in obese patients may promote reflux.
- Avoid eating near bedtime; this allows the stomach to be empty at the time of recumbancy.
- Avoid aggravating factors, including dietary components (i.e. chocolate, fatty foods etc.), cigarettes and alcohol, which decrease LES pressure.
- Avoid medications [i.e. nonsteroidal anti-inflammatory drugs (NSAID), calcium channel blockers] that may decrease LES pressure and delay gastric emptying.

Cytoprotectives

Sucralfate, a basic aluminum salt, exerts a generalized cytoprotective effect (in acidic environment) by enhancing gastroesophageal mucosal defense mechanisms, acting as a barrier to the diffusion of acid, pepsin and bile salts. A safe, well-tolerated drug, effective in relieving symptoms and healing mild esophagitis.

Prokinetic agents

These agents act by increasing LES pressure and by enhancing gastric and esophageal emptying.

Metoclopramide, a dopamine antagonist with cholinomimetic agonist effects, modulates foregut function as described, and is effective at controlling mild GERD. Its use is limited by extrapyramidal side-effects (i.e. dystonias, dyskinesias and parkinsonian symptoms), particularly in the elderly and in children.

Cisapride restores motility throughout the length of the GI tract by enhancing the physiologic release of acetylcholine at the myenteric plexus, without exerting an effect on gastric acid secretion. In addition to increasing LES tone, gastric and duodenal emptying are enhanced by increased contractility and antro-duodenal coordination. Several studies have confirmed the efficacy of this drug (alone or in combination with antacids).

Antacids

1. Silicates. Simple antacids (available over the counter) are clearly useful to reduce gastric acidity, and are widely used for mild GERD. Maximal efficacy requires strict administration (especially in relation to meals), and therefore compliance is a difficulty.

2. H_2-blockers. Cimetidine, ranitidine, famotidine, etc. have all been used widely. Reflux symptoms and healing of esophagitis is seen in 50–60% of patients within 12 weeks of therapy.

3. Proton-pump inhibitors. Proton-pump inhibitors (i.e. omeprazole, lansoprazole) are very effective in treating GERD, with 80–100% improvement of symptoms and healing within 8 weeks of therapy. For patients that respond to therapy, symptoms will return after stopping the drug in the majority of cases. In North America, omeprazole is currently approved for only short-term use, whereas in Europe, many patients currently take this medication long-term. The theoretical concern of carcinogenicity related to long-term acid suppression has not been proven, to date.

Further reading

Sontag SJ. The medical management of reflux esophagitis: role of antacids and acid inhibition. *Gastroenterology Clinics of North America*, 1990; **19:** 683.

Spechler SJ. Comparison of medical and surgical therapy for complicated gastroesophageal reflux disease in veterans. *New England Journal of Medicine*, 1992; **326:** 786.

Tytgat GNJ. Long-term therapy for reflux esophagitis. *New England Journal of Medicine*, 1995; **333:** 1148.

Related topics of interest

HEMOPTYSIS (MASSIVE)

Simon Pickard, Alan G. Casson

Massive hemoptysis is defined as bleeding into the airway that endangers life. There are several quantitative definitions ranging from 100 to >1000 ml blood over 24 hours, with most authors settling on >600 ml over 24 hours. Asphyxiation occurs as the tracheobronchial tree fills with blood; exsanguination is rarely the cause of death.

Etiology

1. Inflammatory lung disease (85%). Tuberculosis accounts for the majority of cases. Bleeding may result from rupture of a Rasmussen aneurysm (false aneurysm of bronchial arteries crossing the wall of a tuberculous cavity), acute exudative lesions (necrosis of small branches of pulmonary arteries or veins), and from erosion of a calcified lymph node into the bronchus (with acute ulceration of bronchial mucosa). The following inflammatory lung diseases have also been linked with massive hemoptysis: (i) Aspergillosis, through undefined mechanisms. (ii) Necrotizing pneumonitis and lung abscess (aspiration and alcoholism), with bleeding secondary to necrosis of pulmonary vasculature. (iii) Cystic fibrosis, through several mechanisms including a dilated tortuous bronchial circulation, bronchopulmonary shunts and pulmonary abscesses.

2. Bronchiectasis with bleeding secondary to proliferation and enlargement of bronchial arteries and precapillary bronchopulmonary anastomoses.

3. Carcinoma. Generally this is an uncommon cause of massive hemoptysis, but it may occur as a result of bronchial artery proliferation (tumor neovascularization).

4. Trauma and bronchovascular fistulae. Results from injury to a major branch of the pulmonary artery (or other thoracic vascular structures) and its associated airway.

5. Pulmonary embolus. Infarction of lung following distal embolization, with resulting necrosis, may result in bronchial artery bleeding. This may be aggravated by anticoagulation.

6. Arterio-venous fistula. This may be a manifestation of hereditary hemorrhagic telangiectasia (Rendu–Osler–Weber syndrome). Bleeding occurs following rupture of thin-walled precapillary pulmonary arterio-venous fistulae, which communicate with the pulmonary vasculature.

7. Cardiac valvular disease. Mitral stenosis may lead to hypertensive rupture of small pulmonary vessels, reversal of blood flow through bronchopulmonary venous connections, and dilation and rupture of submucosal bronchial veins. Embolization from tricuspid valve vegetations may produce pulmonary infarction and hemoptysis.

8. *Iatrogenic.* Secondary to pulmonary artery catheters, anticoagulation, bronchoscopy etc.

Diagnosis

1. *Clinical features.* A complete history is essential to characterize the extent and nature of hemoptysis, and to exclude hematemesis and epistaxis. Details of recent medication should specifically include anticoagulant use. Patients are said to be able to localize the site of bleeding, but this is often unreliable.

2. *Radiography.* Plain X-ray, CT scanning, radionuclide-perfusion scanning and selective bronchial angiography may be used to identify the site and cause of the bleeding.

3. *Bronchoscopy.* Rigid bronchoscopy during active bleeding is essential to maintain the airway, localize and control the site of bleeding and may be diagnostic. Appropiate specimens are taken for microbiology, cytology, etc.

Management

The aims of management are to prevent asphyxiation, to stop ongoing bleeding and to provide definitive treatment of the underlying pathology.

1. *Immediate*
- Position patient bleeding side and head down.
- Oxygen-monitor saturation and/or blood gases.
- Sedatives and antitussives to depress (but not abolish) coughing.
- Large-bore IV access, group and crossmatch.

Rigid bronchoscopy is essential to maintain the airway, to aspirate blood and clot from the tracheobronchial tree, and for ventilation. After localization of the bleeding site, control may be obtained by lavage with ice-cold saline (causes vasospasm). Persistent bleeding is tamponaded by placement of a bronchial balloon blocker and endotracheal intubation. Patients are ventilated (using PEEP), and the bronchoscopy is repeated after 12–24 hours to assess ongoing bleeding, prior to definitive management. Selective intubation, or use of a bronchial blocker, is preferred to a double-lumen endotracheal tube to isolate a lung, unless the latter can be placed expediently.

2. *Definitive management.* Depending on the underlying etiology this may involve the following. (i) Medical therapy with antibiotics, reversal of anticoagulants, etc. (ii) Arterial embolization. Most recent reports suggest that embolization (if

technically possible) is highly successful at controlling bleeding initially. Various rates of relapse or recurrence are reported, and therefore more definitive management may still be required. Occlusion of arteriovenous malformations, using detachable balloons, coiled springs, etc. is now considered to be definitive management (even for large lesions), with few patients now requiring surgical intervention. (iii) Surgical resection may be performed urgently, or after the control of bleeding and following further evaluation of the lesion and patient. (iv) Radiotherapy (external beam or brachytherapy) may be used if a primary or secondary lung tumor is not resectable, or if the patient is not suitable for surgery.

Further reading

Conlan AA. Massive hemoptysis: diagnostic and therapeutic implications. *Surgery Annual*, 1985; **17:** 337.

Jones DK, Davies RJ. Massive hemoptysis. Medical management will usually arrest the bleeding. *British Medical Journal*, 1990; **300:** 889.

Wedzicha JA, Pearson MC. Management of massive hemoptysis. *Respiratory Medicine*, 1990; **84:** 9.

Related topics of interest

HEMOTHORAX

Chris Compeau, Michael R. Johnston

Accumulation of blood in the pleural space most often results from chest trauma, or following iatrogenic intervention (i.e. surgery, thoracentesis and diagnostic needle biopsy procedures). Rare causes include pulmonary embolus, infective processes (i.e. tuberculosis) or neoplasm. Although chest-tube drainage alone is required to manage most cases, thoracotomy may be indicated in selected patients to control ongoing bleeding. Failure to evacuate a hemothorax is a major risk factor for the development of empyema or fibrothorax with a resulting trapped lung.

Etiology

1. *Trauma*
   - Blunt or penetrating injury.
   - Often associated with rib fractures.
   - Source of bleeding commonly intercostal vessels, internal thoracic vessels, lung parenchyma, bronchical arteries, major pulmonary vessels, heart or great vessels.

2. *Iatrogenic*
   - Postoperative. Surgical sources of bleeding after thoracotomy are numerous. However, the following sites are seen most often: inferior pulmonary ligament vessels, from chest-wall adhesions, bronchial vessels or intercostal vessels.
   - Thorcentesis. Lacteration of intercostal vessel.
   - Needle lung biopsy. Unusual with fine-needle aspiration. Incidence increases with use of core-biopsy techniques. Intercostal vessels, pulmonary vessels or tumor may bleed.

3. *Spontaneous pneumothorax.* A rare cause of hemothorax, usually resulting from a tear of a vascular adhesion.

The following conditions commonly produce a bloody effusion but only rarely are they the cause of a frank hemothorax.

4. *Pulmonary embolus.* Bleeding most often occurs following pulmonary infarction (reperfusion of infarcted pulmonary tissue).

5. *Tuberculosis.* A rare cause of significant hemothorax.

6. *Neoplasm*
   - Lung carcinoma with pleural or chest-wall invasion.
   - Metastatic lung or pleural disease.
   - Mesothelioma.

Diagnosis

A high index of suspicion should be maintained following thoracic trauma, especially if associated with respiratory distress. The type, location and extent of the injury need to be considered. Physical signs suggest pleural fluid, confirmed by CXR (upright and lateral decubitus films). Supine trauma chest films (AP) may be difficult to interpret, but may show a hazy lung field secondary to a dependant fluid collection (posteriorly). Thoracentesis is diagnostic. Cell count is generally unhelpful.

Management

1. General. Attention should be directed to ensure that the airway is maintained, along with placement of appropiate monitoring lines, IV access, etc. Blood should be sent for group and crossmatch, clotting parameters and hematocrit analysis. Assessment and management of the patient occur concurrently, and attention should be directed towards identification of associated injuries, or defining the extent of associated pathology.

2. Specific. Specific management involves the placement of a chest tube, preferably 36 F, using the fifth or sixth intercostal space in the mid-axillary line and directing the tube posteriorly. Thoracotomy should be considered in the following circumstances:

- If the initial chest tube output is >1500 ml blood, or >1000 ml with hypotension. If massive bleeding occurs on placing the chest tube, it should be clamped (to tamponade bleeding), and the patient prepared for immediate thoracotomy.
- The ongoing chest tube output is >300 ml/hour for 3 hours.
- If drainage of the hemothorax is inadequate (i.e. a persistent collection is identified radiologically) despite the insertion of a second or third large-bore chest tube.
- Thoracotomy is required to manage associated intrathoracic injuries or pathology.

Thoracoscopic drainage is increasingly reported. Empyema or fibrothorax with trapped lung may result in 10–15% of patients (at least) if a clotted hemothorax remains which can not be evacuated by chest tubes. A CT may be useful to evaluate the extent, location, degree of organization and lung compression associated with the residual hemothorax. This should be treated by early thoracotomy (or thoracoscopy) and drainage, assuming there are no contraindications to general anesthesia. Beyond 4–6 weeks, organization of the clot with development of a fibrothorax requires a decortication.

Further reading

Coselli JS, Mattox KL, Beall AC. Re-evaluation of early evacuation of clotted hemothorax. *American Journal of Surgery*, 1984; **148:** 785.
Meyer DM, Jessen ME, Wait MA, Estera AS. Early evacuation of traumatic retained hemothoraces using thoracoscopy. a prospective, randomized trial. *Annals of Thoracic Surgery*, 1997; **64:** 1396.

Related topics of interest

Chest tubes (p. 42)   Trauma (p. 265)

HIATUS HERNIA

Donna E. Maziak, F. Griff Pearson

The anatomy and physiology of the esophagogastric junction and lower esophageal sphincter, particularly related to dysfunction, remain poorly understood. A hernia is defined as protrusion of a viscus, or part of a viscus, through its normal coverings into an abnormal situation. Herniation of abdominal contents (almost always stomach) through the esophageal hiatus is extremely common. Often this is asymptomatic, and may require no specific therapy. Incarceration, however, may result in complications common to any hernia (i.e. obstruction, volvulus, ulceration, bleeding, perforation, etc.) and as this represents a mechanical problem, is likely to require surgery (i.e. a hiatus hernia repair). Gastroesophageal reflux disease (a functional disorder) may be associated with hiatus herniation. Management of this disorder, medically or by anti-reflux surgery (which may include a hiatus hernia repair), is considered separately.

Classification and pathophysiology

1. Type I (sliding). Axial herniation of the stomach results in the esophagogastric junction lying above the diaphragm. This is thought to predispose to failure of esophagogastric competence, and a sliding hiatus hernia may therefore be associated with GERD.

2. Type II (paraesophageal). Also known as a rolling hernia, as the stomach (or part) herniates through an often enlarged hiatus adjacent to the esophagus (usually anterolaterally) into the mediastinum. As the esophagogastric junction is not displaced, a type II hiatus hernia is generally not associated with reflux. A pure paraesophageal hernia is rare, and is most likely to have a sliding component (type III, below).

3. Type III (combination). A combination of a sliding and paraesophageal hernia.

4. Type IV (complex). Herniation of other abdominal viscera (i.e. colon, omentum, spleen, liver, small bowel), in association with stomach.

Complications

1. Functional. These include GERD and its associations (i.e. esophagitis, bleeding, stricture, aspiration, Barrett's mucosa).

2. Mechanical. These are specific to any hernia. Incarceration results in variable degrees of obstruction of the lower esophagus (i.e. dysphagia) or gastric outlet (i.e. postprandial fullness), and may be intermittent. Volvulus, results from rotation of the herniated stomach along a longitudinal (organoaxial) or transverse (mesenteroaxial) axis. As the herniated stomach enlarges, the mobile greater curvature rotates in the mediastinum (usually to the right side). This may result in the following additional complications.

- Bleeding. Vascular congestion of gastric mucosa may result in iron deficiency anemia. Massive bleeding may result from peptic ulceration.
- Perforation resulting from strangulation and gangrene.
- Impared pulmonary function. Rarely from space occupation, more likely from associated aspiration.

Clinical presentation

A hiatus hernia may be asymptomatic, or present with vague (nonspecific) upper abdominal or respiratory symptoms. A careful history will elicit symptoms of gastroesophageal reflux. Patients may present with symptoms related to the mechanical complications of herniation, including dysphagia, acute chest pain, inability to vomit, postprandial fullness, early satiety, chronic iron deficiency anemia, perforation, hypotension, shock, etc.

Diagnosis

1. Chest X-ray. A CXR may show a retrocardiac air/fluid level, or mediastinal mass.

2. Barium swallow. This should be performed with care, under direct supervision, particularly if obstruction, aspiration or perforation are suspected. Defines foregut anatomy, level of obstruction, position of the stomach and its ability to empty.

3. Endoscopy. This is used to assess the level of the esophagogastric junction, to exclude associated pathology (i.e. tumor) and to assess associated esophagitis or esophageal stricture. This examination may be difficult technically, as the gastric outlet may not be visualized in view of angulation and volvulus of the intrathoracic stomach. Failure to find a bleeding site in the stomach does not rule out a gastric origin for chronic blood loss.

4. Esophageal function studies (manometry, 24-hour pH). These may be useful in selected patients (i.e. sub-acute or nonurgent cases) to assess esophageal function preoperatively.

Management

1. Type I hernia. This type of hernia does not require hiatus hernia repair. Associated gastroesophageal reflux should be managed medically in the first instance. The indications for anti-reflux surgery are discussed elsewhere. The significance of a short esophagus remains controversial. However, this finding remains of critical importance in the appropiate selection of an anti-reflux procedure.

2. Types II, III, IV. Potential complications of herniation suggest that surgical repair (i.e. hiatus hernia repair) is warranted, even if asymptomatic, assuming anesthetic risk is acceptable. Emergency surgery is associated with significantly increased morbidity and mortality, compared with elective repair. The principles of surgery are as follows.

(a) To reduce the hernia and its contents. This may be achieved using an abdominal or left thoracic approach. Early reports have suggested the feasibility of laparoscopy.

(b) To excise the sac and close the hiatus (posteriorly).

(c) To correct any associated pathology (i.e. oversew of a bleeding ulcer, excision of gangrenous viscera).

(d) To fix the stomach in the abdomen. Gastropexy may be achieved in a number of ways:

- By suture of the stomach (lesser curve) posteriorly to the median arcuate ligament (preaortic fascia).
- Suture of the fundus to the diaphragmatic hiatus.
- Using an anterior gastrostomy.

Many surgeons perform a fundoplication concurrently. However, it should be appreciated that this is done in an attempt to prevent recurrent herniation (by providing 'bulk' below the hiatus), rather than as an anti-reflux procedure. It would be logical to perform an anti-reflux procedure in patients who have gastroesophageal reflux disease suspected clinically (if urgent surgery is required) or proven with objective studies (ambulatory 24-hour pH, manometry) if elective repair is performed.

Further reading

Feldman M. Hiatal hernia and gastroesophageal reflux: another attempt to resolve the controversy. *Gastroenterology*, 1993; **105:** 951.

Matthews HR. A proposed classification for hiatal hernia and gastroesophageal reflux. *Diseases of the Esophagus*, 1996; **9:** 1.

Rosati R, Bona S, Fumagalli B. Laparoscopic treatment of paraesophageal and large mixed hiatal hernias. *Surgical Endoscopy*, 1996; **10:** 429.

Sontag SJ, Schnell TG, Miller TQ. The importance of hiatal hernia in reflux esophagitis compared with lower esophageal sphincter pressure of smoking. *Journal of Clinical Gastroenterology*, 1991; **13:** 628.

Williamson WA, Ellis FH, Streitz JM, Shahian DM. Paraesophageal hiatal hernia: is an anti-reflux procedure necessary? *Annals of Thoracic Surgery*, 1993; **56:** 447.

Related topics of interest

LUNG CANCER: CHEMOTHERAPY

Sean Grondin, Michael R. Johnston

Chemotherapy has taken on increased importance in the overall management of NSCLC. Traditionally, it had been reserved for patients with symptomatic Stage IV disease. However, recent clinical trials have evaluated chemotherapy in the neo-adjuvant setting.

Chemotherapeutic agents

Cisplatin, mitomycin C, vindesine, vinblastine and ifosfamide are currently the most active single agents, with response rates >15%. However, single-agent therapy results in a lower response rate and survival time than the combination of two or more agents. Combination chemotherapy may signficantly improve quality of life in responders. Promising new chemotherapeutic agents include docetaxel, paclitaxel, gemcytabine, navelbene, and zeniplatin. Further advances may be made with the administration of biologic-response modifiers (i.e. interferon, interleukin, colony-stimulating factors and labeled monoclonal antibodies). The new metalloproteinase inhibitors and anti-angiogenesis agents are currently undergoing early clinical trials in NSCLC.

Postoperative adjuvant chemotherapy

There are currently no conclusive data to support the use of chemotherapy as a postoperative adjuvant to surgical resection of NSCLC. However, because of systemic failure rates in patients with early-stage NSCLC, ongoing clinical trials are evaluating the efficacy of newer drug combinations (i.e. cisplatin and vinorelbine, taxol and carboplatin) administered postoperatively.

Induction (neoadjuvant) chemotherapy

The rationale for induction chemotherapy is: (i) that a tumor has an intact blood supply (hence better delivery of chemotherapeutic agents) before surgery or radiotherapy; (ii) tumor chemosensitivity may be evaluated for measurable disease; (iii) eradication of micrometastases; and (iv) potentially improved resectability. This approach has been investigated most extensively in patients with Stage IIIA (N2) disease. Patients showing stable disease or an objective response to induction therapy are considered candidates for surgery, which has been shown to be feasible, with minimal morbidity and mortality. An improvement in survival over surgery alone has been noted in several small randomized studies. Reported median survival is about 18 months, with estimated 5-year survival rates of 25–35%. Poor correlation was seen between radiologic (40–70%) and pathologic (15–20%) response. Patients with no evidence of residual tumor in the surgical specimen appeared to have prolonged survival. The use of induction chemotherapy in either Stage IIIA or Stage IIIB disease is still considered experimental and is not advocated outside of a protocol setting.

Concurrent chemoradiotherapy

Certain chemotherapy agents (i.e. cisplatin) are radiosensitizers which accentuate the radiation effect. The optimal sequence for administration of chemotherapy and radiotherapy (i.e. sequentially, concurrently or alternating) has not yet been determined. Potentially, chemoradiotherapy offers both systemic and local control, but is only applicable to patients with good performance status. Randomized studies have shown an improvement in response rates and survival in Stage IIIB and unresectable Stage IIIA NSCLC, however, this approach should not yet be considered as standard practice.

Small cell lung cancer

See 'Small cell lung cancer', p. 224.

Further reading

Einhorn LH. Neoadjuvant and adjuvant trials in non-small cell lung cancer. *Annals of Thoracic Surgery*, 1998; **65:** 208.

Johnson DH. Adjuvant chemotherapy for non-small cell lung cancer. *Chest*, 1994; **106 (Suppl):** 313S.

Natale RB. Experience with new chemotherapeutic agents in non-small cell lung cancer. *Chest*, 1998; **113:** 32S.

Shepherd FA. Induction chemotherapy for locally advanced non-small cell lung cancer. *Annals of Thoracic Surgery*, 1993; **55:** 1585.

Related topics of interest

Lung cancer: radiotherapy (p. 151)
Lung cancer: surgery (p. 154)
Small cell lung cancer (p. 224)

LUNG CANCER: DIAGNOSIS AND STAGING

Sean Grondin, Michael R. Johnston

In a patient with a suspected lung malignancy further investigations are necessary to confirm the clinical impression. Through a series of noninvasive and invasive tests, a tissue diagnosis is secured and the tumor is assessed for both local invasion and distant spread (staging).

Clinical presentation

Symptoms and signs may arise as a result of: (i) local invasion of the primary tumor; (ii) regional spread within the thorax and to the mediastinum; (iii) distant (extrathoracic) metastasis; or (iv) as a result of paraneoplastic syndromes.

1. Primary tumor. Up to 20% of patients with a primary tumor may be asymptomatic. Respiratory symptoms predominate in the majority (>70%) of patients, and may result from central, endobronchial tumor growth (i.e. cough, dyspnoea, unresolved pneumonia, wheeze, hemoptysis) or as a result of a peripheral location (i.e. chest-wall pain, pleural effusion, restrictive dyspnoea, tumor cavitation). It should be noted that coexisting cardiorespiratory disease may mask or mimic these findings.

2. Regional spread. Direct invasion or metastasis to the following intrathoracic or mediastinal structures may result in characteristic symptoms and signs.

- *Pleura.* Pleural effusion (10–15%), resulting in dyspnoea; pleuritic chest pain.
- *Chest wall.* Severe, persistent, localized chest pain results from direct chest-wall invasion.
- *Pericardium.* Malignant pericardial effusion is uncommon at first diagnosis, but is found in up to 35% of patients at autopsy.
- *Superior vena cava.* See 'Superior vena cava syndrome', p. 233.
- *Superior sulcus tumors.* See 'Pancoast tumors', p. 184.
- *Cervical sympathetic nerves.* Horner's syndrome (unilateral enopthalmous, ptosis, meiosis, anhidrosis).
- *Recurrent laryngeal nerve.* Hoarseness, more common with left-sided tumors as a result of the long intrathoracic course of the nerve and its close proximity to mediastinal lymph nodes in the aortopulmonary window.
- *Phrenic nerve.* Paralysis of a hemidiaphragm.
- *Esophagus.* Dysphagia as a result of extrinsic compression (typically enlarged subcarinal nodes), or direct invasion resulting in an esophagobronchial fistula.

3. Distant (extrathoracic) metastasis. Virtually any organ may be involved, with little variation between the four tumor histologies. The most common sites include the adrenals, liver, bone and brain.

4. Paraneoplastic syndromes. These are the distant effects of a tumor (i.e. endocrine, neurologic, skeletal, hematologic, cutaneous) unrelated to metastasis. They are due to the production of one or more biologically active substances (i.e. ACTH, ADH, calcitonin, growth hormone, neurophysins, parathyroid hormone, etc.) and such syndromes are important clinically in up to 10% of patients. Small cell lung cancer is commonly associated with ectopic adrenocorticotropic hormone (ACTH) secretion producing Cushing's syndrome, ectopic vasopressin producing the syndrome of inappropiate antidiuretic hormone (SIADH) and hyponatremia, and the Eaton–Lambert myasthenic syndrome. Squamous cell carcinomas are most commonly associated with ectopic parathyroid hormone-like secretion and hypercalcemia. Anorexia, cachexia, general malaise and low-grade pyrexia are common in lung cancer patients, and may result from tumor necrosis factor, interleuken-1, and prostaglandin production.

Diagnosis

1. History and physical examination

2. Sputum cytology. Standard cytological preparations have not been advantageous in lung cancer early detection studies and have little role in the routine work-up of patients with suspected lung cancer.

3. Chest X-ray. A CXR is the initial diagnostic procedure of choice in patients suspected of having lung cancer. It may help localize the primary lesion (central or peripheral) and detect the presence of mediastinal or hilar adenopathy, pleural effusions or lung consolidation. Characteristic radiologic patterns are seen with each histologic type.

- *Squamous cell carcinoma.* Central location, occasionally cavitating, associated atelectasis, hilar adenopathy.
- *Adenocarcinoma.* Well-defined peripheral nodule, may have chest-wall involvement if large.
- *Large cell tumors.* Large peripheral mass, may cavitate, associated pneumonia and hilar/ mediastinal adenopathy.
- *Small cell.* Bulky mediastinal lymphadenopathy, large central tumors, or rarely a small peripheral tumor.

Chest X-ray has not been effective in the mass screening for lung cancer in high-risk groups.

4. Computed tomography (CT). CT scanning has proved useful for assessing the primary tumor in relation to its size and proximity to adjacent structures, and for planning surgical approaches. This technique provides detailed assessment of the lung parenchyma, and images the diaphragmatic, pericardial, mediastinal and pleural surfaces. However, it is only about 50% accurate in diagnosing tumor invasion into these structures. Mediastinal lymph node size can be accurately measured using CT, thereby influencing the decision on whether to proceed with invasive mediastinal staging. Imaging of the upper abdomen is mandatory so that the entire diaphragmatic recess is visualized along with liver and adrenals (both common sites of lung cancer metastases).

5. *Magnetic resonance imaging (MRI)*. This technique has no advantage over chest CT in the routine diagnosis and staging of lung cancer. However, it is more accurate than CT in assessing tumor invasion into spinal cord, vertebral bodies and brachial plexus (i.e. for Pancoast tumors).

6. *Bronchoscopy*. Performed using either a rigid bronchoscope or, more commonly, a flexible fiberoptic bronchoscope. This allows visualization of up to the third-order bronchus and plays an essential role in the diagnosis, staging and treatement of lung cancer. Using bronchoscopy direct biopsy of endobronchial tumor is often possible. Cytology from saline lavage, bronchial brushing or transbronchial needle aspiration may provide a diagnosis in more peripheral tumors, however, transbronchial biopsy of peripheral tumors under fluoroscopic control provides a tissue specimen, rather than cytology for analysis.

7. *Percutaneous needle biopsy*. Fluoroscopic or CT-guided needle biopsy successfully diagnoses lung cancer with at least 85–90% accuracy, depending on the expertise of the interventional radiologist and pathologist. This technique is indicated in a high-surgical-risk or inoperable patient where other studies have failed to reveal a diagnosis of lung cancer. Biopsies negative for cancer must be considered indeterminate unless a firm histological diagnosis of benignity (i.e. granuloma, hamartoma) can be made. Complications are uncommon, but include pneumonthorax, hemoptysis and bleeding into the pleural space.

Staging NSCLC

Staging NSCLC is accomplished clinically by assessing three distinct aspects of the tumor.

1. *T descriptor*
- Denotes the primary tumor size and growth pattern.
- A T1 tumor is 3 cm or less in diameter and completely surrounded by lung parenchyma.

- T2 designates a tumor greater than 3 cm; or invading visceral pleura; or within a major bronchus (>2 cm distal to the carina); or associated with atelectasis/obstructive pneumonitis that extends to the hilum but not involving the entire lung.
- T3 tumors are any size, with direct invasion of nonvital (i.e. conventionally resectable) structures such as diaphragm, mediastinal pleura, chest wall and pericardium; or tumors within the mainstem bronchus <2 cm distal to the carina (without involving the carina); or associated with atelectasis/obstructive pneumonitis involving the entire lung.
- Tumors of any size that invade vital structures including heart, great vessels, trachea, esophagus and vertebral body are designated T4 and considered unresectable by standard surgical techniques. Malignant pleural effusions, pericardial effusions and satellite nodules within the ipsilateral lobe are also considered to be T4.
- TX: primary tumor can not be assessed; T0: no evidence of tumor; Tis: carcinoma *in situ*.

2. *N descriptor*
- Indicates spread to lymph nodes within the thorax.
- N0 indicates no evidence of nodal metastases.
- N1 nodes reside within the ipsilateral lung parenchyma.
- N2 designation refers to subcarinal nodes and to paratracheal lymph nodes within the mediastinum that are ipsilateral to the lung tumor.
- N3 nodes are those in the mediastinum contralateral to the lung tumor or in either supraclavicular regions.
- NX: regional nodes can not be assessed.

3. *M descriptor*
- Refers to the presence or absence of distant metastasis and must always be considered prior to any therapeutic intervention.
- M0: No distant metastases.
- M1: Distant metastases present.

Stage groupings –
TNM subsets (NSCLC)

TNM subsets provide information about prognosis, allow comparison of outcomes from different clinical series and guide therapy. They have recently been modified to address the wide range of 5-year survivals seen within previous stage groupings (*Table 1*).

Table 1. NSCLC stage groupings and TNM subsets

Stage	TNM subsets
0	Carcinoma *in situ*
IA	T1 N0 M0
IB	T2 N0 M0
IIA	T1 N1 M0
IIB	T2 N1 M0
	T3 N0 M0
IIIA	T3 N1 M0
	T1, T2 or T3 N2 M0
IIIB	Any T4, any N3 M0
IV	Any T, any N M1

Staging investigations

1. Mediastinoscopy/mediastinotomy. Cervical mediastinscopy allows access to paratracheal and subcarinal mediastinal nodes. The procedure involves a small incision in the suprasternal notch, dissection below the pretrachial fascia with direct visualization and biopsy of mediastinal lymph nodes. Anterior medistinotomy, using an incision in the left second interspace is reserved primarily for enlarged nodes or tumor in the left aortopulmonary window region, an area not easily accessed by conventional cervical mediastinoscopy. The accuracy of these procedures is greater than 90%. Major complications occur in fewer than 5% of patients and include bleeding from mediastinal vessels, tracheal or esophageal injury and pneumothorax.

2. Thoracoscopy (VATS). Direct thoracoscopy has been replaced by video-assisted thorascopic surgical (VATS) techniques that may be useful in the diagnosis and staging of some lung cancers. VATS allows access to peripheral lung nodules and the biospy and sampling of mediastinal nodes, especially in the aortopulmonary window. It is most useful for examining the pleural space for evidence of pleural seeding of the tumor.

3. Metastatic work-up. A CT scan of the chest and upper abdomen is essential to evaluate the lung, mediastinum, liver and adrenal glands. In addition a radionuclide bone scan and CT scanning of brain and abdomen are essential in patients with signs or symptoms of metastases to these areas. In the absence of signs or symptoms, the yield from these studies is low and controversy exists on their routine use in patients with lung cancer.

Staging SCLC

See 'Small cell lung cancer', p. 224.

Further reading

Canadian Lung Oncology Group. Investigation for mediastinal disease in patients with apparently operable lung cancer. *Annals of Thoracic Surgery*, 1995; **60:** 1382.

Grover FL. The role of CT and MRI in staging of the mediastinum. *Chest*, 1994; **106 (Suppl.):** 391S.

Kirschner PA. Cervical mediastinoscopy. *Chest Surgery Clinics of North America*, 1996; **6:** 1.

Mountain CF. Revisions in the international system for staging lung cancer. *Chest*, 1997; **111:** 1710.

Mountain CF, Dresler CM. Regional lymph node classification for lung cancer staging. *Chest*, 1997; **111:** 1718.

Shields TW. The significance of ipsilateral mediastinal lymph node metastasis (N2 disease) in non-small cell carcinoma of the lung. *Journal of Thoracic and Cardiovascular Surgery*, 1990; **99:** 48.

Thomas PA. The role of mediastinal staging of lung cancer. *Chest*, 1994; **106 (Suppl.):** 331S.

Related topics of interest

Bronchoscopy (p. 32)
Lung cancer: etiology and pathology (p. 145)
Pancoast tumors (p. 184)
Small cell lung cancer (p. 224)
Video-assisted throracoscopic surgery (p. 275)

LUNG CANCER: ETIOLOGY AND PATHOLOGY

Sean Grondin, Michael R. Johnston

During the past three decades, the incidence of lung cancer has increased significantly in developed countries. Presently, lung cancer is the most common malignancy in men and second only to breast cancer in women. This disease accounts for approximately 25% of all cancer deaths annually in the USA and is the number one cause of cancer death in men and women. Despite recent advances in treatment, the overall 5-year survival for all lung cancer patients is only 13%, primarily due to the advanced stage of the disease at presentation.

Etiology

Smoking

Smoking is the number one risk factor for lung cancer. Based on epidemiologic and experimental studies, it is responsible for about 85% of all lung cancers. The level of risk varies according to the type of tobacco, duration of smoking, amount of tobacco smoked and the tar content of the tobacco. Tobacco smoke is a complex mixture, containing tumor initiators, promotors, cocarcinogens and carcinogens (i.e. nitrosamines and polycyclic aromatic hydrocarbons). Passive smoking is also a risk factor for lung cancer and is estimated to account for approximately 3% of all lung cancers. Passive smokers have been found to have elevated biomarkers of tobacco exposure.

Environmental risk factors

Exposure to radon, asbestos, chromium, silica, nickel and arsenic have all been implicated in lung cancers. Possible risk factors include beryllium, cadmium, diesel exhaust and urban air pollution. The percentage of lung cancers attributable to occuptional factors ranges from 3 to 17%, and smoking and occupational exposure are additive risk factors.

Dietary factors

Dietary factors may either increase (i.e. dietary fat and cholesterol) or decrease lung cancer risk, and epidemiologic studies have demonstrated a protective effect for fruit and vegetable intake. Retinoids (i.e. beta-carotene, a dietary vitamin A precursor) are known to inhibit tumor development and progression experimentally; high dietary intake, and serum level, is associated with decreased lung-cancer incidence.

Preexisting lung disease

A statistically increased risk of lung cancer has been reported in patients with chronic obstructive pulmonary disease and diffuse pulmonary fibrosis. The mechanisms of carcinogenesis in these cases are unclear. Preexisting lung scarring (i.e. from tuberculosis or infarct) was previously thought to be associated with lung carcinogenesis. However, recent studies of scar carcinomas suggest that scarring may be a secondary phenomenon.

Inheritance

An association between lung cancer and positive family history has been described in a limited number of case-controlled studies. The inheritance of a rare autosomal codominant gene, resulting in an earlier age of onset of lung cancer in affected families, has been proposed.

Molecular genetic alterations

Numerous genetic alterations have recently been described in lung cancer. Genetic alterations may be classified as having a positive influence (i.e. oncogenes, such as *ras*, *myc*, *neu*), or a negative, regulatory influence (i.e. tumor suppressor genes, such as *p53*, *Rb*) on cell growth. The relative importance of individual genetic lesions, the sequence of genetic events and the pathways by which altered genes modulate multistep lung carcinogenesis, is unknown.

Pathology

In current practice, lung cancer is conveniently divided into non-small cell lung cancer (NSCLC) and small cell lung cancer (SCLC) because of basic differences in biological behavior, and consequently the therapeutic approach to the two diseases. Malignant epithelial tumors (i.e. carcinomas) of the lung are currently classified histologically, based on features of differentiation and presumed histogenesis (presumed cell of origin), using the WHO scheme. The major types, and key clinicopathologic features, are summarized as follows.

Adenocarcinoma

Histologically, adenocarcinomas show variable degrees of glandular differentiation. Primary lung adenocarcinomas are now the most common cell type, accounting for about 45% of lung cancers. However, differentiation of these from metastatic (secondary) adenocarcinomas may be difficult. Tumors tend to be located in peripheral lung parenchyma, and lymph node metastasis is common. Bronchioloalveolar carcinoma (BAC) is a subtype of adenocarcinoma with a unique growth pattern along the alveolar septae. It often presents as multifocal, synchronous or metachronous lesions, or as diffuse parenchymal disease.

Squamous cell (epidermoid) carcinoma

Histologically, these carcinomas exhibit keratinization (although this varies with differentiation). Approximately 30% of lung malignancies are squamous cell tumors and they tend to be located centrally near the hilum or major bronchi. The carcinoma often has a prominent endobronchial component, with a propensity for local invasion. This cell type is the one most likely to produce malignant cells on sputum cytology.

Large cell (undifferentiated) carcinoma

A precise histologic definition of this carcinoma is controversial. These tumors show an absence of glands or keratinization and account for 5–10% of all lung malignancies. Large cell carcinomas tend to be located peripherally, and poorly differentiated tumors often cavitate. Early metastasis to the mediastinum and brain is common.

Mixed tumor histology Mixed tumor histology is not uncommon, suggesting a common stem-cell origin for lung carcinomas. Therapy in these cases should be directed by the cell type with the worst prognosis.

**Carcinoid and
uncommon lung tumors** • See 'Carcinoid and uncommon lung tumors', p. 39.

Small cell lung cancer • See 'Small cell lung cancer', p. 224.

Further reading

Greenblatt MS, Reddell RR, Harris CC. Carcinogenesis, and cellular and molecular biology of lung cancer. In: Roth JA, Ruckdeschel JC, Weisenburger TH, eds. *Thoracic Oncology*, 2nd edn. Philadelphia: WB Saunders, 1995; 5.

Miller AB. Epidemiology, prevention and prognostic factors, and natural history of lung cancer. *Current Opinions in Oncology*, 1992; **4:** 286.

Roth JA. Biology. In: Pearson FG, Deslauriers J, Ginsberg RJ, Hiebert CA, McKneally MF, Urschel HC, eds. *Thoracic Surgery*. New York: Churchill Livingstone, 1995; 637.

World Health Organization. Histologic typing of lung tumors. *International Histological Classification of Tumors*, 2nd edn. Geneva: World Health Organization, 1981.

Related topics of interest

LUNG CANCER: FOLLOW-UP AND OUTCOME

Sean Grondin, Michael R. Johnston

The overall 5-year survival for all lung cancer patients is 13%. Fifty percent of patients will have advanced disease (Stage IV) at presentation. Most of those cured of their lung cancer will have had surgical resection of their tumor.

Routine follow-up of the lung cancer patient

Typical postoperative follow-up includes history, physical examination and CXR every 3 months for 2 years, every 6 months for the subsequent 3 years and then yearly. Careful follow-up of lung cancer patients permits the early identification of second primary tumors and tumor recurrence, and the accurate assessment of treatment regimens. However, the efficacy (and cost) of close follow-up on survival has recently been questioned. At present there is no place for routine CT scans or MRI in follow-up.

Tumor recurrence

Typically, recurrence is detected within the first 2–3 years following resection and can occur locally, regionally and systemically.

1. Local recurrence. This is defined as a recurrent tumor within the same lung or at the surgical margins. The most common sites are the bronchial stump, and, in T3 tumors, the chest wall. Such tumors should be treated by resection if technically possible or if not, by radiotherapy.

2. Regional recurrence. This signifies recurrence within the mediastinal lymph nodes. Surgery is virtually never indicated and radiotherapy should be considered if the patient is symptomatic.

3. Systemic recurrence. Defined as recurrence in the contralateral lung or at any site outside of the thorax. The treatment options are similar to those for patients who present with Stage IV disease.

Second primary cancers

Long-term survivors of lung cancer are at increased risk of developing second (or multiple) primary tumors of the upper aerodigestive tract (i.e. oropharynx, esophagus, lung). Non-small cell lung cancer is a major cause of late mortality in long-term survivors of small cell cancer. Tumors may develop as a result of field cancerization, where the aerodigestive tract epithelium is exposed to a common carcinogen (i.e. tobacco smoke). Chemoprevention studies are ongoing; agents include retinol, isoretinoin, beta-carotene, vitamin E, folate and selenium.

Results for NSCLC

1. Stage IA, B resected: 60–85% 5-year survival. The best results (80–85% 5-year survival) are seen in patients with T1 N0 bronchioloalveolar carcinoma, and results with squamous carcinoma are significantly better than adenocarcinoma. No adjuvant therapy has been shown to improve survival. Ten to fifteen percent of cured patients will develop a second primary lung cancer.

2. Stage IIA, B resected: 40–60% 5-year survival. No difference in survival has been demonstrated between cell types. Adjuvant radiation therapy decreases incidence of local recurrence but does not improve overall survival. Most patients who relapse are found to have systemic metastases.

3. Stage IIIA: 10–40% 5-year survival. Patients with completely resected T3 N1 do signficantly better (30–40% 5-year survival) than those with N2 disease. No difference in survival between cell types has been shown. Patients receiving induction therapy followed by surgical resection who are found to have had a complete pathological response (no tumor demonstrated in the surgical specimen) probably have improved survival over other therapies for IIIA (N2) disease.

4. Stage IIIB: <10% 5-year survival. There is a possible survival advantage for selected patients with completely resected T4 N0 tumors but experience is small and surgery is high-risk. Concurrent chemoradiotherapy prolongs median survival by months in good performance patients, although treatment is usually aimed at palliating symptoms.

5. Stage IV: <5% 5-year survival. All therapies are palliative, and if the patient has no symptoms, no therapy is an acceptable choice.

Results in SCLC

See 'Small cell lung cancer', p. 224.

1. Extensive disease: <5% 5-year survival. Median survival 8–12 months.

2. Limited disease: <20% 5-year survival. Median survival 12–15 months.

3. Very limited disease: ~25% 5-year survival. This catergory includes the unusual patient with resected Stage I or Stage II disease by the TNM classification.

Further reading

Ginsberg RJ. Follow-up supervision after resection for lung cancer. In: Delarue NC, Eschapasse H, eds. *International Trends in General Thoracic Surgery*, Vol. 1. Philadelphia: WB Saunders, 1985.

Rosengart TK, Martini N, Ghosn P, Burt M. Multiple primary lung carcinomas: prognosis and treatment. *Annals of Thoracic Surgery*, 1991; **52:** 773.

Tockman M, Erozan Y, Gupta P, Piantadosi S, Mulshine JL, Ruckdeschel JC. The early detection of second primary lung cancers by sputum immunostaining. *Chest* 1994; **106 (Suppl.):** 385S.

Related topics of interest

LUNG CANCER: RADIOTHERAPY

Sean Grondin, Michael R. Johnston

In lung cancer management, radiotherapy can be utilized as a primary treatment, as an adjuvant to surgery or chemotherapy, or as palliative therapy to alleviate symptoms. Treatment is usually delivered by external beam. However, brachytherapy techniques are becoming more popular for selected indications. Increasingly, radiotherapy is administered (sequentially, concurrently or alternating) with chemotherapy, which may increase tumoricidal response without a corresponding increase in normal tissue toxicity.

Primary treatment with radical external beam radiation

Patients with early-stage (I or II) NSCLC, who either refuse surgery or are medically unfit for surgery, are treated with radical radiotherapy (at least 65 Gy to the primary tumor in daily fractions of 1.8–2.0 Gy). Local failure rates for this treatment are reported at 30% for T1 tumors and 70% for T2 tumors. Five-year survival rates range from 5 to 40%, the difference being attributable to differences in technique and pretherapy staging. Accelerated fractions, hyperfractionation and 3-dimensional therapy are new approaches that are currently under investigation. Additional prognostic factors for radical radiotherapy include patient performance status, pulmonary reserve and tumor biology.

Adjuvant radiotherapy

Several trials have evaluated postoperative radiotherapy after complete resection of N1 or N2 disease, and for patients with positive bronchial resection margins. Although locoregional recurrence rates are reduced with this approach, this has not translated into improved overall survival. As most treatment failures are at distant sites, recent clinical trials have evaluated adjuvant chemoradiotherapy. The results have, to date, been inconclusive. A feasibility trial is ongoing to evaluate VATS wedge resection and adjuvant radiotherapy for high-risk patients with T1 N0 NSCLC.

Preoperative radiotherapy

Classically, preoperative radiotherapy (30 Gy in 10 days) has been used to treat T3 Pancoast tumors prior to surgical resection. Postoperative radiation therapy has been given inconsistently. Data supporting this approach are anecdotal, as a randomized study would be difficult to perform as there are relatively few patients with Pancoast tumors. A current multicenter Phase II trials are evaluating preoperative chemoradiotherapy. Although preoperative radiotherapy is used at some centers in an attempt to decrease the incidence of local chest wall recurrence after *en bloc* surgical resection of NSCLC, supportive data for this approach are lacking.

Palliative radiotherapy	This technique offers good symptomatic relief for malignant bronchial obstruction and hemoptysis from endobronchial tumor. It has a high success rate in relieving pain from bone metastases and improving neurologic symptoms from brain metastases. Radiotherapy may also be used to treat patients with symptomatic SVC syndrome secondary to locally invasive NSCLC. See 'Superior vena cava syndrome', p. 232.
Brachytherapy	This involves the treatment of a tumor by the direct application of a radioactive source and therefore, permits the delivery of a localized, high dose of radiotherapy. The radioactive source may be placed interstitially (directly into the tumor) or intracavitary (within the airway using a bronchoscopically placed afterloading catheter). The technique is useful in the palliation of endobronchial lesions. Its superiority to external-beam radiation has not been established despite decreased toxicity.

Complications

1. *Esophagitis*
- Transiently experienced by up to 50% of patients.
- Usually starts within 2 weeks of initiating therapy, and lasts until 2 weeks after.

2. *Pneumonitis*
- Present to some degree radiographically in all patients; clinically significant in 5%.
- Patients undergoing chemoradiotherapy may be at increased risk of pulmonary toxicity.
- Severity of symptoms (i.e. dry cough, low-grade fever) are related to the volume of lung irradiated.
- May progress to productive cough (pink sputum) and respiratory failure.
- Differential diagnosis includes viral or bacterial pneumonia, recurrent tumor, or lymphangitic spread.

3. *Pericarditis*
- May be associated with pericardial effusion and myocarditis.
- Usually resolves spontaneously.

4. *Myelitis*
- Neural (and cord) injury is related to increasing radiation fraction.

Further reading

Einhorn LH. Neoadjuvant and adjuvant trials in non-small cell lung cancer. *Annals of Thoracic Surgery*, 1998; **65:** 208.

Greenberger JS, Bahri S, Jett JR, Belani CP, Kalend A, Epperly M. Considerations for optimizing radiation therapy for non-small cell lung cancer. *Chest*, 1998; **113:** 46S.

Hazuka MBO, Turrisi A. The evolving role of radiation therapy in the treatment of locally advanced lung cancer. *Seminars in Oncology*, 1993; **20:** 174.

Weisenburger TH. Effects of postoperative mediastinal radiation on completely resected stage II and III epidermoid cancer of the lung: LCSG 773. *Chest* 1994; **106 (Suppl.):** 297S.

Related topics of interest

LUNG CANCER: SURGERY

Sean Grondin, Michael R. Johnston

Surgery is the most effective treatment for early-stage (I and II) NSCLC, assuming the primary tumor can be resected completely, and that the perioperative risk is low. Approximately 25% of patients have resectable disease at the time of presentation. Surgery may also be indicated for selected patients with advanced stage (III, IV) NSCLC, and for a limited number of patients with SCLC.

Lung cancer diagnosis and staging
See 'Lung cancer: diagnosis and staging', p. 139.

Preoperative evaluation
See 'Preoperative assessment for thoracic surgery', p. 212.

Surgical principles
A complete resection of the primary tumor and its intrapulmonary lymphatics is essential. This is achieved by an anatomic resection, most commonly lobectomy or pneumonectomy. Segmentectomy may be appropriate in selected situations but has a high incidence of local recurrence. An *en bloc* or extended resection is indicated for selected patients with locally advanced tumors, who are without evidence of regional lymph node metastases. At surgery, the tumor should not be visualized or transgressed to avoid tumor spillage. Intraoperative frozen section should be performed to confirm negative resection margins (i.e. bronchus, vessels, adjacent structures) and to ensure a complete resection. The intraoperative staging of lymph nodes should be performed. Formal dissection of nodal stations provides more accurate staging than sampling alone. Survival benefit, or reduction in local recurrence, following extensive lymph node dissection is controversial.

Stage I and II NSCLC
Lobectomy (or bilobectomy, pneumonectomy) is the surgical treatment of choice in these patients. Lesser resections (i.e. wedge, segmentectomy) should be reserved for high-risk patients who will not tolerate lobectomy. An increased incidence of locoregional recurrence (10–15%) is seen in patients undergoing lesser resection. Radiation therapy may be offered to patients who refuse surgery or are medically inoperable (i.e. cardiac disease). See 'Lung cancer: radiotherapy', p. 151.

Locally advanced NSCLC (T3, 4)
Selected patients with locally advanced primary tumors (T3, 4) are amenable to surgical resection alone, or surgery following induction therapies. A complete surgical resection is required for long-term survival, and an extended, or bronchoplastic, procedure is often necessary. These tumors include T3 chest-wall tumors, T3 Pancoast tumors, T3 disease involving the mediastinum or mainstem bronchus, and selected T4 tumors (usually detected at thoracotomy and judged to be completely

resected) involving the heart (usually left atrium), trachea and carina, esophagus or vertebral body. Survival rates in this group decrease significantly with lymph node involvement and it is essential to exclude distant metastases with this stage of disease.

N2 NSCLC

At present, the management of N2 disease is controversial, and subject to clinical trials. The incidental finding of N2 disease at thoracotomy (i.e. microscopic disease, squamous histology, limited to one lymph node station, completely resected) may be associated with 5-year survival rates of up to 30%. However, this is applicable to only a small number of patients with N2 disease. Preoperatively identified N2 disease (i.e. by mediastinoscopy) is generally associated with poor 5-year survival (<6%) with surgery alone and patients with N2 disease are at increased risk of having distant metastases. Currently, combined modality therapy is considered to be optimal (vs. surgery or radiotherapy alone), although the combination and sequence of modalities has not been determined. Preoperative radiotherapy has no advantage, but current clinical trials are evaluating induction chemotherapy, followed by surgery or radiotherapy.

N3 NSCLC

Contralateral mediastinal lymph node metastases are considered by most surgeons to be an absolute contraindication to surgery, as long-term survival is dismal. A limited number of studies have evaluated induction chemoradiotherapy followed by radical surgical excision and extended lymph node resection (using sternotomy or clamshell incisions). Although a few survivors are reported (suggesting the need for further clinical trials), this approach is unlikely to become routine clinical practice.

Solitary metastasis (M1)

1. Brain. This is a frequent site of metastatic disease in patients with resected NSCLC, and patients with untreated brain metastases have a median survival of 3 months. Radiation therapy is the treatment of choice for multiple metastases, while solitary lesions are managed by surgery provided that the brain metastasis is completely resected, all thoracic disease is controlled and no distant metastases are identified. Overall 5-year survival may approach 20% in this highly selected group of patients.

2. Lung. Solitary pulmonary metastases are occasionally seen, but differentiation from second primary tumors may be difficult. In the absence of regional nodal (or distant) metastases, resection should be performed.

3. Adrenal gland. Solitary adrenal metastases are identified with increasing frequency because of CT scanning of the upper abdomen. Although resection of solitary lesions is reported, long-term survival is unknown.

4. Other sites. Solitary metastases are rarely identified at various distant sites (i.e. bone, liver, muscle, skin). Anecdotal long-term survival is reported following complete resection of a solitary metastasis, provided that the primary tumor is controlled and no additional metastases are identified.

Surgical options for NSCLC

1. Wedge/segmental resection. Indications include peripheral lung tumors (<3 cm) in patients with poor pulmonary reserve, metachronous or synchronous lesions and diagnostic biopsy. Recurrence rates are higher, and survival reduced, when compared with lobectomy.

2. Lobectomy/bilobectomy. This includes complete resection of hilar (N1) lymph nodes draining the primary tumor, and allows preservation of lung function while still providing adequate tumor margins. Complete resection must be ensured by obtaining a frozen section on the bronchial margin. Re-resection to a negative margin, use of a bronchoplastic procedure, or conversion to pneumonectomy should be considered if positive margins are identified operatively. Mortality rates should be less than 3%.

3. Pneumonectomy. Accounts for about 20% of all lung resections, and is indicated when tumor invades hilar structures, such as mainstem bronchus or main pulmonary artery. It may also be indicated for tumors crossing the oblique fissure, or for lymph node involvement along the mainstem bronchus, proximal to the upper lobe takeoff. The procedure results in considerable loss of lung parenchyma with possible significant chronic respiratory impairment.

The morbidity is higher than for lobectomy (i.e. atrial arrhythmias, bronchial stump leaks, respiratory insufficiency), and mortality rates are 6–8%.

4. Extended pulmonary resections. See 'Extended pulmonary resection', p. 117.

5. Bronchoplastic procedures. See 'Bronchoplastic (sleeve) procedures', p. 26.

Video-assisted thoracoscopic surgery (VATS)

See 'Video-assisted thoracoscopic surgery', p. 275. Currently, routine application of VATS for definitive treatment of lung cancer is not recommended. It may be used for wedge resection of peripheral tumors in high-risk surgical patients, provided surgical principles are adhered to.

Palliation

1. Laser therapy. This should not be considered definitive therapy for lung cancer, but is useful in palliating exophytic tumors of the trachea and bronchi, to restore the airway or prior to definitive therapy. It may be effective for *in situ* carcinoma in conjunction with photodynamic therapy.

2. Palliative resections. Noncurative pulmonary resection may occasionally be indicated in the following situations, in the hope of improving a patient's quality of life:

- Unrelenting sepsis from a lung abscess, caused by bronchial obstruction by tumor.
- Massive hemoptysis where death from asphyxiation or exsanguination is imminent.

Further reading

Pearson FG. Current status of surgical resection for lung cancer. *Chest*, 1994; **106 (Suppl.):** 337S.
Rubinstein LV, Ginsberg RJ. Lobectomy versus limited resection in T1N0 non-small cell lung cancer. *Annals of Thoracic Surgery*, 1996; **62:** 1249.
Van Raemdonck DE, Schneider A, Ginsberg RJ. Surgical treatment for higher stage non-small cell lung cancer. *Annals of Thoracic Surgery*, 1992; **54:** 999.

Related topics of interest

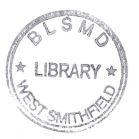

LUNG TRANSPLANTATION

Ziv Gamliel

Since the first successful lung transplant in 1983, over 4000 lungs have been transplanted worldwide. Improved selection criteria (donor and recipient), better immunosuppression regimens, technical advances and postoperative management have contributed to current survival rates approaching 70% at 2 years. However, lack of organ donors, postoperative infection and chronic rejection continue to limit pulmonary transplantation.

Donor considerations

Donor selection criteria

- Age <55 years.
- No history of pulmonary disease.
- Normal serial CXR.
- Adequate gas exchange (PaO_2 >300 on 100% O_2 and PEEP 5 cmH$_2$O).
- Normal bronchoscopic examination.
- Negative serologic screen for hepatitis B and HIV.
- ABO blood group matched to recipient.
- Size approximately matched to recipient.

Donor operation

The superior vena cava (SVC), inferior vena cava (IVC) and ascending aorta are encircled and the donor is heparinized. A pulmonary artery flush cannula is inserted just proximal to the main bifurcation. Venous inflow is eliminated by occluding or dividing the SVC and IVC. With the lungs still ventilated, the pulmonary artery is flushed with 3 l of iced (1–4°C) modified Euro-Collins solution (containing 3% glucose and 4 mEq/l MgSO$_4$) vented via the amputated tip of the left atrial appendage. Topical ice is applied on the lungs and cold effluent is allowed to collect in the pleural spaces. The heart is extracted taking care to preserve a rim of atrial muscle on the pulmonary veins. The lungs are extracted as a single block, mobilizing from below, dividing the trachea using a stapler with the lungs in moderate inflation. The lungs are separated by dividing the posterior wall of the left atrial cuff in the middle, dividing the pulmonary artery at its bifurcation and stapling the proximal left mainstem bronchus with a linear cutter stapler to maintain inflation. The lungs are then transported in iced saline (1–4°C). Immediately prior to implantation, and while still in their ice bath, the lungs are prepared by trimming away excess pericardium and mediastinal fat, dissecting the atrial cuff aound the pulmonary veins and trimming the length of the dissected pulmonary artery.

Recipient considerations

Disease indications

1. Obstructive pulmonary disease

(a) Emphysema

- Most common indication for transplantation.
- Patients typically are on oxygen but have a stable course on the waiting list.
- Consider single or bilateral transplantation.

(b) Alpha-1 antitrypsin deficiency

- Generally younger patients with less cardiovascular disease.

2. Septic lung disease: cystic fibrosis

- Most common inherited disorder among white patients.
- Most patients will die before age 40 without transplantation.
- Up to one-third of patients may die on waiting list.
- Bilateral transplant required because both septic lungs must be removed.

3. Fibrotic lung disease: pulmonary fibrosis

- One of the less common indications for transplanation.
- May be associated with some degree of pulmonary hypertension.
- Patients often deteriorate rapidly on the waiting list.

4. Pulmonary vascular disease

(a) Primary pulmonary hypertension

- High risk of sudden death, and highest death rate on the waiting list.

(b) Eisenmenger's syndrome

- Single lung transplantation.
- Repair cardiac defect.
- An alternative to heart–lung transplantation.

Recipient selection criteria

- Clinically and physiologically severe disease.
- Substantial limitation in activities of daily living.
- Medical therapy ineffective or unavailable.
- Limited life expectancy (12–24 months), age up to 60 years.
- Adequate cardiac function without significant coronary artery disease.
- Ambulatory with rehabilitation potential.
- Acceptable nutritional status.
- Satisfactory psychosocial profile and emotional-support system.

Recipient operation

The decision to perform a single- or double-lung transplant is based on the status of the remaining lung. Therefore, single-lung transplantation is appropiate for patients with COPD and pulmonary fibrosis, whereas double-lung transplantation should be used for patients with cystic fibrosis or bronchiectasis. The most appropiate procedure for patients with pulmonary hypertension is controversial, although most centers prefer double-lung procedures. Bilateral transplants are performed using bilateral fourth intercostal space anterolateral thoracotomies joined by a transverse sternotomy (clamshell incision). Unilateral transplants are performed using a posterolateral thoracotomy. The side with least pulmonary function is transplanted first. Cardiopulmonary bypass may be used to facilitate the procedure if pulmonary hypertension is present.

Postoperative management

1. Physiologic support. Most patients are extubated by pressure support or intermittent mandatory ventilation (IMV) wean within 24–48 hours postoperatively. Pulmonary hypertensives may require sedation and paralysis for 48–72 hours before weaning can begin. PEEP should be kept to a minimum in patients undergoing single-lung transplantation for emphysema to avoid hyperinflation of the more compliant native lung. Fluids are administered judiciously, monitoring the pulmonary capillary wedge pressure. Early diuresis facilitates weaning.

2. Sepsis prophylaxis. Broad-spectrum antibiotic prophylaxis is used perioperatively. Specific antipseudomonal coverage is guided by preoperative sputum cultures in patients with cystic fibrosis, who may also receive aerosolized colistin or tobramycin. Donor cultures are also reviewed. *Pneumocytis carinii* prophylaxis with cotrimoxazole is virtually completely effective, and although fungal prophylaxis with fluconazale is not used routinely, it may be warranted by the finding of *Candida* in donor cultures. Acyclovir is routinely used for prophylaxis against herpes simplex viruses. This is changed to gancyclovir if either the donor or the recipient is found to be seropositive for cytomegalovirus.

3. Immunosuppression. Chronic immunosuppression usually consists of cyclosporine (maintained to levels of 250–300 ng/ml), azathioprine and prednisone. Prednisone is reduced as much as possible to prevent long-term complications of steriod use. Cyclosporine is initiated by continuous infusion in the first few postoperative hours after satisfactory urine output is ensured. Blood levels are initially maintained to levels between 350 and 400 ng/ml. Azathioprine may be given immediately at a dose of 1–2 mg/kg/day. The initial IV dose can be directly converted to oral dosing. The leukocyte count must be closely monitored. After the initial high dose of methylprednisolone (500 mg) administered intraoperatively prior to lung reperfusion, patients are maintained with

0.5–1 mg/kg/day. Oral prednisone is initiated after the first few days and is slowly tapered to low levels. Cytolytic therapy with antithymocyte globulin in the early postoperative period has been used to reduce the incidence of acute rejection but its efficacy remains unproven. This therapy may actually be associated with an increased incidence of cytomegalovirus infection. Trials are currently underway to evaluate the efficacy and safety of this practice

Surveillance

Routine surveillance with pulmonary function tests, CXR, bronchoscopy, bronchoalveolar lavage cultures and transbronchial biopsies is performed at prescribed intervals and whenever clinically warranted. Most patients will develop acute rejection within the first 3 weeks of transplantation, and this is characterized by dyspnea, low-grade fever, leukocytosis, hypoxemia and perihilar interstitial infiltrates. In such instances, rejection must be differentiated from infection. Suspected acute rejection is effectively treated with high-dose methylprednisolone, 500–1000 mg. In cases of acute rejection, clinical and radiologic improvement will usually be seen within 8–12 hours, prompting the administration of two additional daily doses. Chronic rejection remains difficult to treat and is manifested by obliterative bronchiolitis. Chronic allograft dysfunction in the form of a steady decline in FEV_1 has been termed bronchiolitis obliterans syndrome. Augmented immunosuppression will result in improvement in the occasional patient, but this can usually only retard the progression of chronic rejection and diminishing FEV_1.

Postoperative complications

1. Early graft dysfunction. This complication occurs in approximately 20% of patients and may represent unsuspected pathology in the donor lungs (i.e. aspiration, infection, contusion). Management of the condition usually includes increased PEEP and diuresis, and, in certain cases, consideration may be given to use of inhaled nitric oxide.

2. Infection. This is usually bacterial, but may be viral or fungal.

- *Bacterial.* Rule out *Burkholderia cepacia* in patients with cystic fibrosis.
- *Viral.* Cytomegalovirus infection is most likely in donor-negative recipient-positive patients. Presence of cytomegalovirus in bronchoalveolar lavage specimen is not necessarily indicative of infection.
- *Fungal.* Usually *Aspergillus.*

3. Pleural space complications
(a) Pneumothorax
- Rarely a result of airway dehiscence.

- Often due to size discrepency in recipients with chest cavities larger than the donor lungs (in which case this can be ignored).
(b) Pleural effusions may be due to size mismatch or underlying parenchymal disease.
(c) Empyema is unusual in transplant patients but may occur in association with prolonged air leaks.

4. Airway complications. The donor bronchus relies on collateral pulmonary flow for blood supply during the first few days following transplantation. Impaired healing may result in bronchopleural fistula (requiring a chest tube) or stricture (requiring stenting or dilatation).

5. Rejection. Transbronchial biopsy is the preferred diagnostic modality for rejection. Acute rejection early postoperatively occurs in nearly all patients but is rarely a significant clinical problem. Chronic rejection is the most common underlying cause of late death and has no effective therapy. It is manifested by development of bronchiolitis obliterans with a steady fall in FEV_1. The progression of chronic rejection may be slowed or arrested with increased immunosuppression. Selected patients with advanced chronic rejection may be considered for retransplantation.

Results

1. Operative mortality. Early mortality in lung transplantation ranges between 8 and 21% and is most commonly due to sepsis or organ failure. Operative mortality is higher in bilateral transplants, transplants for primary pulmonary hypertension and transplants for cystic fibrosis colonized by *B. cepacia.*

2. Late mortality. The main causes of late death are sepsis and bronchiolitis obliterans. Overall 5-year survival in lung transplantation approaches 60% and is longer for bilateral transplants than single transplants.

3. Functional results. Most patients enjoy normal exercise tolerance without supplemental oxygen within 6–8 weeks. Early functional assessment reveals little difference between single and bilateral transplants, although bilateral transplantation offers significant late advantage in preservation of FEV_1 due to higher reserve.

Further reading

Cooper JD, Pearson FG, Patterson GA. Technique of successful lung transplantation in humans. *Journal of Thoracic and Cardiovascular Surgery*, 1987; **93:** 173.
DeHoyas AL, Patterson GA, Maurer JR. Pulmonary transplantation: early and late results. *Journal of Thoracic and Cardiovascular Surgery*, 1992; **103:** 295.

Khaghani A, Al-Kattan KM, Tadjkarimi S, Banner N, Yacoub M. Early experience with single lung transplantation for emphysema with simultaneous volume reduction of the contralateral lung. *European Journal of Cardiothoracic Surgery*, 1997; **11:** 604.

Kshettry VR, Kroshus TJ, Hertz MI, Hunter DW, Shumway SJ, Bolman RM. Early and late airway complications after lung transplantation: incidence and management. *Annals of Thoracic Surgery*, 1997; **63:** 1576.

Patterson GA, Cooper JD, Goldman B. Technique of successful clinical double-lung transplantation. *Annals of Thoracic Surgery*, 1988; **45:** 626.

Sundaresan S, Cooper JD. Lung transplantation. *Annals of Thoracic Surgery*, 1998; **65:** 293.

Sundaresan S, Trachiotis GD, Aoe M. Donor lung procurement: assessment and operative technique. *Annals of Thoracic Surgery*, 1993; **56:** 1409.

Unruh HW. Lung preservation and lung injury. *Chest Surgery Clinics of North America*, 1995; **5:** 91.

Related topics of interest

LUNG VOLUME REDUCTION SURGERY

Alan G. Casson

Lung volume reduction surgery (LVRS) has recently emerged as a palliative surgical procedure for patients with end-stage emphysema. This has been facilitated by improvements in preoperative evaluation, advances in surgical technique and improved postoperative management. Removal of diseased and functionless lung is believed to improve the function of the remaining (less diseased) lung by: (i) increasing elastic recoil pressure, leading to increased expiratory flow rates; (ii) decreasing the degree of hyperinflation, resulting in improved chest-wall and diaphragmatic mechanics; and (iii) decreasing the work of breathing and improving alveolar gas exchange.

Patient selection

There are currently no absolute preoperative selection criteria to define patients who will benefit from LVRS, and the following guidelines are evolving.

- Patients should be dyspneic, with impaired activities of daily living and quality of life, despite maximal medical therapy or pulmonary rehabilitation.
- Age <75 years.
- Radiographic evidence of generalized emphysema, with regional heterogeneity (target areas for resection), and no bullae >5 cm diameter.
- Air trapping and hyperinflation, with a total lung capacity more than 125% of predicted.
- FEV_1 <30% of predicted.
- $PaCO_2$ <50 mmHg; PaO_2 >40 mmHg on room air.
- No significant associated illness (i.e. coronary artery disease, pulmonary hypertension).
- Steroid dosage <15 mg/day.

Preoperative investigations

- History and physical examination.
- Objective quality of life, activity assessment.
- Pulmonary function studies, including exercise testing.
- Arterial blood-gas analysis.
- Chest X-ray.
- CT scanning (high-resolution).
- Radionuclide ventilation/perfusion scanning.
- Cardiac investigations (EKG, echocardiography, catheterization) as indicated.

Surgical techniques

- Double-lumen endotracheal anesthesia is required.
- Incisions include:
    Median sternotomy (bilateral LVRS)
    Unilateral VATS LVRS
    Bilateral VATS LVRS (single or staged procedures).
- Generally 20–30% of each upper lobe (50–75 g lung tissue) is resected conforming to the lung contour. The

Results

mechanically stapled tissues may be buttressed with bovine pericardium to reduce air leakage. Other target areas for resection are identified by preoperative scanning, but clinical judgement is required at the time of surgery.

- Patients are extubated immediately following surgery. Chest tubes are not connected to suction.

Experience from single centers suggests that LVRS may be performed with mortality rates below 10%. VATS LVRS may be associated with less morbidity, but no randomized studies have been reported, to date. At 1-year postoperatively, approximately 75% of patients appear to have considerable improvement (subjectively and objectively); however, 15% appear to show little change from their preoperative status. Current trials are attempting to address patient selection for LVRS, the role of pulmonary rehabilitation and the long-term results of LVRS.

Further reading

Cooper J, Trulock E, Triantafillou A. Bilateral pneumectomy (volume reduction) for chronic obstructive pulmonary disease. *Journal of Thoracic and Cardiovascular Surgery*, 1995; **109:** 106.

Fein AM, Branman SS, Casaburi R. Lung volume reduction surgery. *American Journal of Respiratory Critical Care Medicine*, 1996; **154:** 1151.

Kotoloff RM, Tino G, Bavaria JE. Bilateral lung volume reduction surgery for advanced emphysema: a comparison of median sternotomy and thoracoscopic approaches. *Chest*, 1996; **110:** 1399.

Krucylak PF. Lung volume reduction surgery. *Annals of Thoracic Surgery*, 1997; **64:** 1514.

McKenna RJ, Brenner M, Fischel RJ. Should lung volume reduction for emphysema be unilateral or bilateral? *Journal of Thoracic and Cardiovascular Surgery*, 1996; **112:** 1331.

Naunheim KS, Ferguson MK. The current status of lung volume reduction operations for emphysema. *Annals of Thoracic Surgery*, 1996; **62:** 601.

Sciurba FC, Rogers RM, Keenan RJ. Improvement in pulmonary function and elastic recoil after lung volume reduction surgery for diffuse emphysema. *New England Journal of Medicine*, 1996; **334:** 1095.

Yusen RD, Lefrak SS. Evaluation of patients with emphysema for lung volume reduction surgery. *Seminars in Thoracic and Cardiovascular Surgery*, 1996; **8:** 83.

Related topics of interest

MECHANICAL VENTILATION

Fang Gao

The purpose of mechanical ventilation is to apply an external source to do some or all of the work of breathing in situations where the patient is unable to achieve adequate gas exchange.

Indications

1. Deficient gas exchange. Progressive hypoxia [PaO_2 <60 mmHg (8 kPa)] or hypercapnia [$PaCO_2$ >60 mmHg (8 kPa)].

2. Increased work of breathing. Characterized by increasing respiratory rate and decreasing tidal volume (VT <3 ml/kg).

3. Impaired consciousness

4. Following long or complicated surgical procedures. Used to maintain stable respiratory function following the administration of large fluid volumes, excessive blood loss or when there is ongoing intrathoracic bleeding from a diffuse coagulopathy.

Causes of respiratory failure

- Respiratory center depression (i.e. anesthetic drugs, opioids, intracranial pathology).
- Peripheral neuromuscular disorders (i.e. Guillain–Barré syndrome, myasthenia gravis, spinal cord pathology, muscle relaxants).
- Chest-wall defects (i.e. trauma, chest wall resection).
- Reduced alveolar ventilation (i.e. lung or pleural disease, obesity).
- Pulmonary vascular disease (i.e. pulmonary embolus, cardiac failure, ARDS).
- High CO_2 production (i.e. sepsis, burn injury, severe agitation).

Modes of ventilation

Full or partial ventilatory support can be provided by the following.

1. Controlled mandatory ventilation (CMV)
- Fixed ventilation for defined time intervals.
- No provision for spontaneous ventilatory effort.
- Generally limited to intraoperative and immediate postoperative ventilation.

2. Assist control mode. Acts like CMV in the absence of spontaneous breathing. However, when the patient takes a spontaneous breath, the ventilator is triggered to reach a preset level of ventilation.

3. *Intermittent mandatory ventilation (IMV) and synchronized IMV (SIMV).* A mandatory rate of ventilation is preset, but patients are free to breath spontaneoulsy between set ventilator breaths. Mandatory breaths may be synchronized with the patient's spontaneous efforts (SIMV). The advantages of this system (over CMV) are better gas distribution, a lower mean airway pressure, less hemodynamic disturbance, less sedation is required, and weaning is easier.

4. *Pressure support ventilation (PSV).* A preset inspiratory pressure is added to the ventilator circuit during inspiration in spontaneously breathing patients.

Setting up the mechanical ventilator

- Ensure the airway is secure.
- Ensure adequate sedation, opioids and/or muscle relaxants.
- Initial settings: FiO_2 0.5–1.0; V_T 10–12 ml/kg; RR 10–12/min; I:E ratio 1:2; peak pressure <40 cmH$_2$O; PEEP 2–5 cmH$_2$O.
- These settings are adjusted to achieve optimal gas exchange in response to blood-gas measurements. Alterations in FiO_2 and PEEP will alter PaO_2; alterations in V_T and RR will alter $PaCO_2$. Prolonged expiration (i.e. I:E = 1:3) is useful in patients with COPD; prolonged inspiration (i.e. I:E = 1:1 or 2:1) is useful in patients with ARDS.

Weaning

Successful weaning depends on the patient's general condition, central respiratory drive, respiratory muscle strength, nutritional status, any preexisting lung disease and the duration of ventilation. Weaning is likely to be successful when the following have been achieved:

- Recovery from the primary illness.
- Optimization of general medical conditions.
- PaO_2 >60 mmHg (8 kPa) on FiO_2 <0.4.
- $PaCO_2$ <45 mmHg (6 kPa) in non-COPD patients.
- RR <30/min; V_T >5 ml/kg.
- Vital capacity >10 ml/kg; minute volume <10 l/min.

Technique
- SIMV: the set mandatory rate is gradually reduced as the spontaneous rate increases.
- PSV: positive pressure is added to each breath.
- CPAP (continuous positive airway pressure): to prevent microatelectasis.
- Flow by (high gas flow through the circuit to keep inspiratory valve open): to decrease the work of breathing.

Complications

During positive pressure ventilation, the normal subatmospheric intrathoracic pressure during spontaneous ventilation is replaced by positive intrathoracic pressure which may cause detrimental changes in cardiac and respiratory physiology.

1. Cardiovascular. Reduced venous return and increased pulmonary vascular resistance contribute to reduced cardiac output. These complications can be minimized by reducing airway pressures, avoiding high PEEP, avoiding prolonged inspiratory times and maintaining circulating blood volume.

2. Respiratory
- V/Q mismatch; FRC reduction.
- Barotrauma and tension pneumothorax. Minimized by avoiding high V_T, high PEEP and high airway pressures.
- Disuse atrophy of respiratory muscles.

3. Renal. The release of ADH, renin and vasopressin leads to water retention and reduced urine output.

4. Cerebral. A reduced $PaCO_2$ results in vasoconstriction and reduced intracranial pressure.

5. Acid–base disturbance
- Respiratory alkalosis: K^+, Mg^{2+}, and ionized Ca^{2+} reduced; systemic vasoconstriction.
- Respiratory acidosis: systemic vasodilation, arrhythmias.

6. Nosocomial infection. Endotracheal intubation bypasses the body's normal defense, heat and moisture exchange mechanisms.

Continuous positive airway pressure

CPAP is the addition of positive pressure (2.5–10 cmH$_2$O) during expiration in a spontaneously breathing patient via: (i) a tight fitting face mask, (ii) a nasal mask, or (iii) the expiratory limb of a T-piece breathing circuit. In order to achieve CPAP it is necessary to keep the inspiratory valve open with the inspired air–oxygen supply at a flow rate greater than the patient's peak inspiratory flow, or with a large reservoir bag in the inspiratory circuit. CPAP is indicated in: (i) hypoxemia (increases FRC, reduces V/Q mismatch), (ii) left ventricular failure (reduces venous return). This technique should be used with caution in patients with COPD (as the alveolar-to-mouth pressure gradient is reduced). Complications of CPAP include the risk of aspiration, reduced cardiac output, hypercarbia and increased intracranial pressure.

Positive end expiratory pressure

- The addition of positive pressure (usually <10 cmH$_2$O) during the expiratory cycle of mechanical ventilation.
- Indications and complications are similar to CPAP.
- Physiologic PEEP (2–3 cmH$_2$O) is provided normally by a closed larynx.
- Auto-PEEP (intrinsic PEEP, air-trapping). Reduced expiratory time in patients with COPD, results in air-trapping, increased airway pressures and hypercarbia.

High-frequency ventilation (HPV)

- High-frequency positive pressure ventilation (HFPPV).
- High-frequency jet ventilation (HFJV).
- High-frequency oscillation (HFO).

HPV is defined as ventilation at a frequency of more than four times the normal rate, with V_T = 1–3 ml/kg to maintain normocarbia. The mechanisms of improved gas exchange are not elucidated fully, however, increased turbulence and convective mixing, particularly at bronchial bifurcations, may contribute. Advantages over conventional ventilation include improved cardiovascular stability and improved ventilation when the airway is disrupted (i.e. trauma, operative, bronchopleural fistula). Disadvantages include reduced humidification, CO_2 retention, monitoring ventilation and increased driving pressures.

High-frequency jet ventilation
- The most commonly used HFV mode in clinical practice.
- Indications include laryngeal or tracheobronchial surgery, bronchopleural fistula, ARDS.
- A jet of gas, which entrains further gas by the Venturi effect, is delivered at high velocity through a cannula or a jet tracheal tube.
- Usual settings are: driving pressure 1–2 bar (760–1520 mmHg); RR 100–200/min; I:E 1:2–1:3.

Further reading

Kalia P, Webster NR. Conventional ventilation and weaning. New modes of respiratory support. In: Goldhill DR, Withington PS, eds. *Textbook of Intensive Care*. London: Chapman Hall Medical, 1997; 401.

Slutsky AS. Consensus conference on mechanical ventilation. Parts I and II. *Intensive Care Medicine*, 1994; **20:** 64 (Part I), 150 (Part II).

Related topics of interest

Adult respiratory distress syndrome (p. 5)
Anesthesia for thoracic surgery (p. 8)

MEDIASTINUM AND MEDIASTINAL MASSES

Gail Darling

A wide range of mediastinal lesions may present to the general thoracic surgeon for evaluation. Although a surgical approach was previously recommended for virtually all mediastinal lesions, recent advances in imaging, needle-aspiration biopsy techniques and cytopathology can now prevent inappropiate thoracotomies. However, a thorough understanding of the anatomy of the mediastinum, the wide differential diagnosis of mediastinal lesions and an organized approach are essential for accurate diagnosis and management.

Anatomy

The mediastinum is defined as the space between the thoracic inlet and the diaphragm, between the right and left pleural surfaces, which extends from the inner aspect of the sternum to the vertebral column. It is subdivided (arbitrarily) into compartments (i.e. superior, inferior, anterior, middle and posterior), and although there is some overlap, most mediastinal masses tend to occur in a given compartment. Although several classifications have been proposed, the simplest, which corresponds to that used by radiologists to describe the location of mediastinal masses, is based on the lateral CXR.

1. Anterior. Bounded by the posterior table of the sternum (anteriorly) and the pericardium (posteriorly). The anterior compartment is often grouped with the *superior* compartment (i.e. above an imaginary line between the manubriosternal junction and the T4/5 interspace). The normal *anterosuperior* compartment contains thymus, lymph nodes and fat.

2. Middle. This compartment contains the heart and pericardium, superior and inferior vena cavae, ascending aorta and arch, the branches of the arch, the brachiocephalic veins, main pulmonary arteries and veins, phrenic and vagus nerves, trachea and main bronchi, lymph nodes and fat.

3. Posterior. This compartment extends from the pericardium to the posterior chest wall (including the paravertebral gutters) and contains the esophagus, descending aorta, azygous and hemiazygous veins, thoracic duct, sympathetic chain and lymph nodes.

Mediastinal masses and cysts

Primary mediastinal masses and cysts are uncommon and the incidence varies with age (children vs. adults). There has also been a change in incidence reported, with an increasing diagnosis of lymphoreticular and thymic lesions. The most common primary mediastinal lesions are: neurogenic tumors (19%), lymphoma (16%), bronchogenic and pericardial cysts (14%), germ-cell tumors (13%), thymoma (12%) and thyroid lesions (6%). Metastatic lung cancer, infections and other inflammatory conditions are more common than primary mediastinal lesions.

Differential diagnosis of a mediastinal mass

1. *Anterosuperior mediastinum*
- Thymic tumor or cyst.
- Substernal thyroid or neoplasm.
- Germ-cell tumors.
- Lymphoma.
- Lymphadenopathy: metastatic cancer, reactive, infectious (i.e. tuberculosis, fungal), sarcoidosis, Castleman's disease.
- Parathyroid tumors or cysts.

2. *Middle mediastinum*
- Lymphadenopathy.
- Vascular: aortic aneurysm; anomalies of the great vessels.
- Pericardial cyst, or diverticulum.
- Bronchogenic cyst.
- Tracheal tumors.
- Parathyroid tumors or cysts.
- Neural tumors of the phrenic, vagus, sympathetic nerves.

3. *Posterior mediastinum*
- Neurogenic tumors (benign and malignant): peripheral intercostal nerves (neurofibroma, neurilemmoma, neurofibrosarcoma); sympathetic ganglia; ganglioneuroma, neuroblastoma); paraganglia (phaeochromocytoma, paraganglioma).
- Meningocoele.
- Esophageal tumors, diverticulae, duplication cysts.
- Hiatus hernia.
- Thoracic duct cysts, cystic hygroma (lymphangioma).
- Extramedullary hematopoesis.
- Vertebral chordoma.
- Paravertebral abscess (tuberculous).

Clinical presentation

Almost half of patients are asymptomatic and have a normal physical examination. Symptoms and signs depend on the etiology and location of the lesion. Symptomatic lesions are more likely to have a malignant etiology, as are lesions in children.

1. *Symptoms*
- Local: pain (chest or back), dyspnea, cough, dysphagia, etc.
- Systemic: nonspecific fever, malaise, weight loss, night sweats, etc.

2. *Signs*
- Local: cervical lymphadenopathy, facial and/or arm swelling, tracheal deviation.

	• General: testicular masses, hepatosplenomegaly, muscle weakness.

Diagnosis

1. *Laboratory investigations*
   - CBC: anemia, leukocytosis, thrombocytopenia.
   - Lactate dehydrogenase (LDH): elevated in lymphomas, seminomas – also a guide to therapeutic response.
   - β-human chorionic gonadotrophin (β-HCG): may be increased in seminomas. Negative markers do not guarantee a benign diagnosis.
   - α-fetoprotein: indicates a nonseminatomatous component of a germ-cell tumor; normal in pure seminomas.
   - Alkaline phosphatase and calcium: may be altered with parathyroid tumors.
   - Urine metanephrines; VMA; screening of catecholamines for phaeochromocytomas.

2. *Radiology*
   - Chest X-ray.
   - CT scanning with IV contrast.
   - MRI for neurogenic or vascular lesions.
   - Angiography for vascular lesions.
   - Barium swallow for posterior mediastinal masses.
   - Radionuclide scintigraphy for suspected thyroid, or parathyroid masses.
   - Gallium scan in lymphoma.

3. *Biopsy*
   - Fine-needle aspiration biopsy. Accuracy depends on the skill of the interventional radiologist and interpretation by a cytopathologist. Recent immunohistochemical and molecular pathologic techniques now permit accurate classification of lymphomas from limited tissue specimens. A histologic diagnosis may be made from a core of tissue obtained using a larger gauge, or cutting, needle.
   - Mediastinoscopy is particularly useful for biopsing superior or middle mediastinal masses in a paratracheal location.
   - Anterior mediastinotomy is now rarely necessary because of core needle biopsies.
   - VATS is useful for anterior and posterior mediastinal lesions that abut the pleural space.
   - Bronchoscopy is useful in hilar or peritracheal lymphadenopathy or whenever there is a concomitant lung lesion. Trans-bronchial lung biopsy is the procedure of choice in suspected sarcoidosis.
   - Esophogoscopy should be performed for dysphagia or any mass in close proximity to the esophagus.

Management **(general principles)**	• Exclude vascular and congenital lesions. • Differentiate solid vs. cystic lesions. • Obtain a definitive tissue diagnosis. Do not rely on frozen section. • Differentiate primary vs. secondary (i.e. metastatic) tumors. • Assess resectable vs. locally advanced disease.
Thymoma	See 'Thymoma', p. 244.
Neurogenic tumors	• Most common posterior medistinal tumors. • Asymptomatic unless large, invasive, or with extension through the intervertebral foramen into the spinal canal (dumbbell tumor), or the rare pheochromocytoma. • Assuming minimal anesthetic risk, tumors should be excised. • Intrathoracic disease only: thoracotomy or VATS for selected small tumors. • Dumbbell tumors: evaluate with MRI. May require a combined approach (single or staged procedures) with neurosurgeon. Laminectomy and intraspinal dissection is performed initially to prevent cord injury or intraspinal hemorrhage. • Neuroblastoma: primary therapy is chemo/radiotherapy. • Phaeochromocytoma: preoperative α/β blockade, followed by excision. • Paragangliomas: may invade vascular structures (i.e. aorta, heart).
Germ-cell tumors	The anterior mediastinum is the most common site of extragonadal germ-cell tumors. These tumors commonly affect males aged 20–35 years, and investigations should include serum markers and testicular examination with ultrasound. *1. Teratoma.* Markers negative, encapsulated tumors should be excised. Complete resection is associated with excellent prognosis. *2. Seminoma.* Combination chemotherapy (cisplatin, bleomycin, etoposide, vinblastine) and large volume radiotherapy is the primary management. Surgical excision of small (< 3 cm) residual mediastinal masses may occasionally be required. *3. Nonseminomatous* • Embryonal, endodermal sinus (yolk sac), choriocarcinoma, mixed tumor histology. • Elevated markers (β-HCG, α-fetoprotein, LDH) are found in >90% of patients. • Tissue diagnosis is preferable, but therapy may be initiated on the basis of elevated markers alone.

- Management is primarily cisplatin-based chemotherapy, with 50% 5-year survival.
- Residual masses (i.e. benign teratomas, nongerm-cell tumor elements, fibrosis) may require resection since they often slowly enlarge and cause compressive symptoms; markers must have normalized following chemotherapy.
- Salvage chemotherapy is given to patients with residual malignant tumor; prognosis is poor.

Lymphoma

The mediastinum may be involved by lymphoma of any type (Hodgkin's, 60–90%; nonHodgkin's, 20–40%), generally as part of widespread disease; rarely as the only site. Ninety percent of mediastinal lymphomas have lymphoblastic (Hodgkin's) or diffuse large cell (nonHodgkin's) histology, and the majority of lymphoma patients are symptomatic (local, systemic). Management of the disease depends on an accurate tissue diagnosis, obtained by either needle biopsy or by surgical biopsy. Chemotherapy is the mainstay of treatment although radiotherapy or bone-marrow transplantation may be used depending on the stage of the disease and the patient's response to chemotherapy. Surgery may also be used to rebiopsy or excise a residual or nonresponding mass, or to manage any complications of chemoradiotherapy (i.e. pericarditis, pleural effusions).

Bronchogenic cysts

Enlargement of cysts, development of symptoms (cough, dyspnea), and to establish a definitive diagnosis are the principal indications for surgical excision, assuming minimal anesthetic risk.

Enteric cysts

Surgical excision is generally recommended.

Pericardial cysts

An accurate diagnosis can be made by CT scan, echocardiography or needle aspiration if technically feasible. Excision is required only to obtain a tissue diagnosis or if the patient is symptomatic.

Substernal goiter

An anterosuperior mediastinal mass, where >50% of the thyroid is below the thoracic inlet. Respiratory compromise (sudden or chronic with tracheomalacia), dysphagia, SVC obstruction or hyperthyroidism are indications for excision. Large goiters may be removed safely using a neck (collar) incision. Excision of true ectopic thyroid tissue (thoracic vascular supply), posterior mediastinal extention or malignancy may require thoracotomy.

Further reading

Kohman LJ. Approach to the diagnosis and staging of mediastinal masses. *Chest*, 1993; **103** (Suppl.): 328S.

Strollo DC, Rosado-de-Christenson ML, Jett JR. Primary mediastinal tumors. *Chest*, 1997; **112:** 1344.

Walsh GL. General principles and surgical considerations in the management of mediastinal masses. In: Roth JA, Ruckdeschel JC, Weisenburger TH, eds. *Thoracic Oncology*, 2nd edn. Philadelphia: WB Saunders, 1995; 445.

Related topics of interest

Congenital bronchopulmonary anomalies (p. 56)
Thymoma (p. 244)
Video-assisted thoracoscopic surgery (p. 275)

MESOTHELIOMA

Chris Compeau, Michael R. Johnston

Pleural mesotheliomas are relatively rare tumors arising from the mesothelial lining of the lung. There are localized and diffuse forms. The latter are locally aggressive tumors that metastasize late in the clinical course. Management of mesothelioma is generally dictated by the clinical stage of disease and the biology of the tumor.

Localized mesothelioma

- Well-defined encapsulated tumors.
- Not associated with asbestos exposure.
- Benign and malignant variants.

Clinical presentation
- Often an asymptomatic mass, discovered incidentally on CXR.
- Symptoms include cough, chest pain and dyspnea.
- Rarely hypoglycemia, due to secretion of an insulin-like peptide.

Treatment
- Complete surgical resection, if possible.
- Survival is directly related to completeness of resection.
- Long-term outcome unpredictable.

Diffuse mesothelioma

Always malignant, diffuse mesotheliomas are associated with asbestos exposure (amphibole fibers, especially chrysolite). The latency period between exposure and the disease is over 20 years. Other risk factors include radiation exposure, and exposure to other naturally occuring or man-made fibers (straight, narrow) that are taken up by pulmonary lymphatics or pass directly into the lung parenchyma. Smoking is not a risk factor.

Clinical presentation
Dyspnea, chest-wall pain and weight loss are the most common symptoms although patients with locally advanced disease may have a palpable chest-wall mass. Other nonspecific symptoms including weakness, anorexia and fever are seen in up to 25% of patients. Although paraneoplastic syndromes are uncommon, thrombocytosis occurs in up to 40% of patients. Radiographic (i.e. CXR, CT, MRI) appearances include pleural effusions, pleural thickening and contraction of the hemithorax. Mediastinal lymph nodes and distant disease are seen with advanced tumors.

Diagnosis
- Thoracentesis.
- Pleural needle biopsy – tissue sample often insufficient.
- Thoracoscopy and pleural biopsy.

- Open pleural biopsy (with or without decortication).
- Note the propensity of mesothelioma to seed the biopsy tract.

Histology
- Epithelial, sarcomatoid and mixed subtypes.
- Easily confused with metastatic adenocarcinoma.
- Electron microscopy and immunohistochemistry help secure a diagnosis.

Staging

Several staging systems have been proposed for diffuse mesothelioma. Elements of staging include: the presence or absence of tumor invasion into the adjacent chest wall, diaphragm or mediastinal structures; mediastinal lymph-node involvement; and distant metastases. Favorable prognostic factors for this disease are: epithelial histologic type, the absence of chest pain and a good performance status.

Treatment

The choice of therapy is often individualized according to the location and extent of the tumor, stage and performance status of the patient. Response to all therapies is generally poor, although for selected patients, surgery provides a slight improvement in survival.

1. Radiation
- Used to palliate symptomatic chest-wall or mediastinal involvement.
- High-dose radiation of the hemithorax is too toxic.
- Often used in conjunction with surgery or chemotherapy.
- Local control disappointing.

2. Chemotherapy. Many clinical trials have evaluated a variety of chemotherapeutic agents (both alone and in combination) administered either systemically or locally. However, response rates are generally disappointing.

3. Immunotherapy. Promising preliminary response rates are reported with interferon.

4. Surgery
(a) Thoracoscopy and talc pleurodesis
- Thoracoscopy may be used to obtain pleural biopsies.
- A palliative procedure only, appropriate if the pleural effusion is symptomatic and the underlying lung is expandable.
(b) Pleurectomy and decortication
- May be technically difficult.
- Air leaks are common postoperatively.
- Palliative benefit only.
(c) Extrapleural pneumonectomy
- *En bloc* resection of pleura, lung and ipsilateral hemidiaphragm and pericardium.
- Applicable in only 20–25% of patients.

- Operative mortality 5–15%.
- Median survival approximately 1 year, with complete resection.

5. *Combined modality therapy.* This technique involves surgery in combination with radiotherapy and/or chemotherapy to improve disease-free and overall survival. Ongoing randomized clinical trials are limited by the relatively small patient numbers, and the current lack of active agents for this disease.

Further reading

Campbell DB. Malignant mesothelioma. *Annals of Thoracic Surgery*, 1997; **63:** 1503.
Pass HI. Contemporary approaches in the investigation and treatment of malignant pleural mesothelioma. *Chest Surgery Clinics of North America*, 1994; **4:** 497.
Rusch VW, Piantadosi S, Holmes EC. The role of extrapleural pneumonectomy in malignant pleural mesothelioma. *Journal of Thoracic and Cardiovascular Surgery*, 1991; **102:** 1.
Rusch VW, Venkatraman E. The importance of surgical staging in the treatment of malignant pleural mesothelioma. *Journal of Thoracic and Cardiovascular Surgery*, 1996; **111:** 815.
Sugarbaker DJ, Norberto JJ. Multimodality management of malignant pleural mesothelioma. *Chest*, 1998; **113 (Suppl.):** 61S.

Related topics of interest

MYCOTIC INFECTIONS

Simon Pickard, Alan G. Casson

With improved techniques for diagnosis, pulmonary mycotic infections are increasingly recognized in clinical practice, especially in immunosuppressed patients. Surgery may be required for diagnosis, to treat disease resistant to medical therapy, or to manage complications. This section will address general principles related to diagnosis and therapy, and summarize key pulmonary features of selected fungal infections.

Diagnosis

A firm diagnosis can only be established after demonstrating the fungus in body tissues or fluids. Successful culture of the fungus depends on the method of collection. Fresh samples should be delivered to the laboratory as soon as possible after sterile collection, and prolonged incubation may occasionally be required. The highest diagnostic yield for a pulmonary infection is obtained using bronchoalveolar lavage, however, sputum collection, transbronchial biopsy, lymph node biopsy or lung biopsy (VATS or open) may occasionally be required. The involvement of extrapulmonary sites (i.e. blood, joint fluid, mucous membrane biopsy) may establish the diagnosis also. Immunologic changes in the host may suggest a presumptive diagnosis, to enable treatment of life-threatening infection prior to the identification of the organism, and to follow the course of the disease. IgM antibodies appear early after infection and disappear by 6 months. IgG antibodies appear later, peak at 2–3 months, and may persist for years. The direct detection of specific fungal antigens (i.e. *Cryptococcus* polysaccharide capsular antigen by latex agglutination) indicates an active infection.

Management

1. Medical therapy. Remains the mainstay of treatment. The main anti-fungal agents are:
- Amphotericin B. This binds to ergosterol (in fungal cell membranes) causing leakage of cellular contents. Given IV or intrathecally. Dose limited by renal toxicity.
- Ketoconazole. Inhibits cytochrome P450-dependent enzymes; prevents fungal cell-wall construction. Active orally with a wide spectrum of activity; minimal toxicity.
- Itraconazole, fluconazole. Greater specificity against fungal-P450-mediated reactions. Wide range of activity (itraconazole vs. *Aspergillus*; fluconazole vs. *Candida*); low toxicity.

2. Surgery. Surgery may be required to treat disease resistant to medical therapy, including: persistent cavitary disease and complications (i.e. hemoptysis, broncholithiasis, granulomatous fistulae, fibrosing mediastinitis).

Specific infections

1. Aspergillosis. A ubiquitous organism found naturally in soil or as a commensal in the oral cavity. May present as:

- Bronchitic aspergillosis. A form of hypersensitivity. Usually responds to steroids without need for anti-fungal agents.
- Invasive aspergillosis. Presents in debilitated, immunosuppressed patients as pneumonia, pulmonary infarction or generalized sepsis. Associated with high mortality rates, requiring aggressive therapy with itraconazole.
- Aspergilloma. Colonization of cavities (i.e. post tuberculous) within lung parenchyma. Surgical resection may be indicated for localized disease or severe hemoptysis. Recently, interventional radiologic techniques have been employed successfully to instill anti-fungal agents directly through indwelling catheters, or using embolization techniques (i.e. coils) to control hemoptysis.

2. Candida. An opportunistic infective agent which can cause mucocutaneous (i.e. oral, esophageal) or systemic (any organ) infection. Severe debilitating disease, immunosuppression, and prolonged use of antibiotics may predispose to systemic candidiasis, which is treated by systemic therapy with amphotericin B. Mortality remains generally high.

3. Histoplasmosis. A common fungal infection in the USA, predominantly along the Mississippi River valley. Inhaled spores may be asymptomatic, or lead to minimally infective symptoms in the majority of patients. Pneumonia may occur in patients with preexisting pulmonary disease, and the onset of chronic cough, hemoptysis, dyspnoea and pyrexia suggests the development of chronic cavitating disease. Mediastinal involvement (i.e. fibrosing mediastinitis, pericarditis) may lead to further symptoms, including SVC compression. Medical treatment is required initially, but surgery may be required for chronic cavitary disease or complications.

4. Coccidiomycosis. Endemic in south west USA and Mexico. Young children are usually asymptomatic or have minimal pulmonary symptoms. Adults with a first exposure are at risk for pulmonary infection or systemic disease. Skin lesions (i.e. erythema nodosum, erythema multiforme, generalized macules) are associated with the development of an immune response and may be prognostic. An association with arthralgia is known as acute valley fever. As resolution is common, most patients do not require therapy. Five percent will develop bronchiectasis, pulmonary nodules, cavitary disease or abscesses, and may require surgery.

5. *Blastomycosis.* Endemic in the south eastern USA, where spores are found in the soil. Inhalation may lead to pulmonary infection in young male adults. The acute form appears radiologically as patchy lower lobe infiltrates, which resolve over 3 months. Chronic pulmonary blastomycosis has a fibronodular appearance in the upper lobes, with smooth-walled cavities. The skin and musculoskeletal system may also be affected, particularly in chronic disease. Rib involvement is pathognomonic. Treatment is initially medical, although late relapse is not uncommon. Surgery may be required to control bronchopleural fistulae, or to drain empyemas or abscess cavities.

Further reading

Chatzimichalis A, Massard G, Kessler R, Barsotti P, Claudon B, Ojard-Chillet J, Wihlm JM. Bronchopulmonary aspergilloma: a reapprasal. *Annals of Thoracic Surgery*, 1998; **65:** 927.

Pomerantz M. Surgery for pulmonary infections with mycobacterium other than tuberculosis (MOTT). *Chest Surgery Clinics of North America*, 1993; **3:** 737.

Salerno CT, Ouyang DW, Pederson TS, Larson DM, Shake JP, Johnson EM, Maddaus MA. Surgical therapy for pulmonary aspergillosis in immunocompromised patients. *Annals of Thoracic Surgery*, 1998; **65:** 1410.

Related topics of interest

OCCULT LUNG CANCER

Alan G. Casson

Fewer than 1% of patients with lung cancer will have disease that is not detected radiographically. Such patients with occult lung carcinoma may be a challenge to manage, and careful evaluation is essential.

Clinical presentation

1. History and examination. Generally asymptomatic, but may present with hemoptysis or nonspecific symptoms. Patients may be enrolled in early lung cancer detection or surveillance programs. Physical examination should focus on the head and neck region.

2. Radiography. Plain films and CT scanning (high resolution) usually show normal lung fields, although incidental abnormalities may be detected.

Diagnosis

1. Sputum cytology. Malignant cells in sputum may arise from tumors of any part of the upper aerodigestive tract. The diagnostic yield depends on sputum production, tumor size (large), location (central), histology (squamous), methods of collection, and the expertise of the cytopathologist. An induced sputum using inhaled normal saline delivered by an ultrasonic nebulizer provides the best noninvasive means of sampling lower airway secretions. This is usually followed by collecting sputum each morning for the next 3 days. The poorest yield is obtained from small peripheral adenocarcinomas. Sputum cytology may also allow, premalignant dysplastic cells to be diagnosed. Immunocytochemistry, using monoclonal antibodies against tumor-associated markers, may improve the diagnostic accuracy of this technique.

2. Panendoscopy, esophagogastroscopy. This is performed under general anesthesia to exclude upper aerodigestive tract tumors.

3. Bronchoscopy. A careful diagnostic bronchoscopy is performed, using a flexible fiberoptic bronchoscope, to visualize the tracheobronchial mucosa. A pediatric bronchoscope is useful to examine more peripheral bronchopulmonary segments. Any mucosal lesions identified are biopsied for histologic examination. The accuracy of detection of small mucosal lesions using bronchoscopy may be enhanced by laser-induced fluorescence techniques. Washings and brushings are taken from each segmental bronchus in an attempt to localize the site of malignancy. Care should be taken to avoid cross-contamination and to label specimens correctly. If selective sampling reveals malignant cells in a segmental bronchus, washings and brushings should be repeated and the malignancy confirmed before convening therapy. If no malignant cells are found, reassessment is warranted within 3 months. The timing of further surveillance is uncertain.

Stage

TX N0 M0. An occult carcinoma with bronchopulmonary secretions containing malignant cells but without other evidence of the primary tumor or regional lymph node or distant metastases.

Management

Following localization of the occult carcinoma, the treatment of choice is surgical resection, according to the established principles of lung cancer management. This is most often a lobectomy, although a pneumonectomy may be required for central lesions. Long-term survival following surgical resection is over 80% (at 5-years). Patients with an occult tumor may be at increased risk of multiple primary tumors of the upper aerodigestive tract, and therefore surveillance at 6–12 monthly intervals is recommended. Photodynamic therapy has been shown to be effective at eradicating mucosal disease, but the long-term outcome of this treatment is not known. At present this should be reserved for patients who are prohibitive operative candidates.

Further reading

Cortese DA, Pairolero PC, Bergstralh EJ. Roentgenographically occult lung cancer: a ten year experience. *Journal of Thoracic and Cardiovascular Surgery*, 1983; **86**: 373.

Related topics of interest

Bronchoscopy (p. 32)
Lung cancer: diagnosis and staging (p. 139)

PANCOAST TUMORS

Sean Grondin, Michael R. Johnston

A superior sulcus tumor (Pancoast, 1932) was originally reported as an apical lung cancer that, as a result of local invasion, was associated with Horner's syndrome, radiologic destruction of ribs, pain and atrophy of the hand muscles (Pancoast syndrome). This description has been extended to include apical lung tumors locally invading any thoracic inlet structure (i.e. ribs, thoracic vertebrae, brachial plexus, roots of the lower cervical/upper thoracic nerves, sympathetic chain/stellate ganglion, subclavian vein/artery), producing the severe pain and Horner's syndrome characteristic of Pancoast's syndrome. Rarely, other invasive pulmonary lesions (i.e. aspergilloma) may result in a Pancoast syndrome.

Clinical presentation

Pain localized to the shoulder (upper arm or neck), secondary to chest wall invasion and destruction of the ribs, is the commonest symptom (>50% patients). This symptom may have been attributed to musculoskeletal lesions of the neck (i.e. cervical osteoarthritis) or shoulder (i.e. bursitis), resulting in a delayed diagnosis. Symptoms also include numbness and weakness of the arm and hand, resulting from invasion of the lower branches (C8, T1) of the brachial plexus. Horner's syndrome (pupillary constriction, ptosis of the upper eyelid, sinking in of the eyeball, anhydrosis and flushing of the affected side of the face), secondary to invasion of the thoracic sympathetic trunk at the stellate ganglion, is found in 30% of patients. Symptoms related to the underlying lung malignancy, are variably reported by 20–80% of patients, and may include significant weight loss. Additional symptoms (generally <10% of patients) related to local tumor invasion may include paraplegia (cord compression), hoarseness (recurrent laryngeal nerve paresis) and SVC syndrome.

Diagnosis and staging

1. Radiology. Plain CXR usually demonstrates asymmetry at the lung apex (above the clavicles). This may be very subtle (and missed), or attributed to technique or pleural thickening. Apical lordotic or oblique films are often suggested, but are usually unhelpful. An elevated hemidiaphragm suggests phrenic nerve involvement. Bone destruction (ribs, vertebrae) may be seen on the plain film, cervical spine tomography or suggested by increased uptake on a radionuclide bone scan. As with lung cancers generally, CT scanning (chest and neck) defines the relationship of the primary tumor to local structures and may be helpful in planning therapy. However, assessment of direct invasion (tumor/normal interface) may not be accurate. CT will also demonstrate mediastinal node enlargement and distant metastases. MRI (thin section coronal and saggital T1-weighted imaging of the superior sulcus) has shown increased accuracy for assessment of local invasion (T-stage), compared with CT. MRI is also particularly useful for evaluating the extention of tumor into the spinal canal, cord compression and vertebral body invasion. Additional imaging studies (i.e. angiography, myelography) may be useful in selected patients.

2. Bronchoscopy. Fiberoptic bronchoscopy (even with brushings and washings) is reported to be diagnostic in only 30% of patients.

3. Needle aspiration. Fine needle (or core) biopsy of the primary lesion, under radiologic (fluoroscopy or CT) guidance, will provide a tissue (histologic or cytologic) diagnosis in most (>95%) patients.

4. Scalene node biopsy, mediastinoscopy. Accurate nodal staging is essential to the management of patients with superior sulcus tumors (as for any lung cancer). This may be achieved by invasive techniques (i.e. mediastinoscopy or scalene node biopsy).

Management

As these tumors were considered inoperable (and incurable) because of their relative inaccessibility and the extent of local invasion, only palliative radiation therapy was attempted initially. Subsequently, surgical excision was shown to be feasable, especially following preoperative radiotherapy. This approach became generally accepted as the standard therapy, based on a large nonrandomized series (and several smaller series) from individual centers, but has recently been questioned. Although satisfactory local control may be achieved by radical surgery, with considerable palliative benefit, most patients develop systemic disease. This underlies the rationale for recent clinical trials evaluating multimodality therapy for these tumors. Patients with inoperable disease (technically unresectable, medically unfit, metastases) are best managed with palliative radiotherapy (external beam or brachytherapy) or chemoradiotherapy to relieve pain.

Surgery

All patients should undergo thorough staging (to exclude distant metastases), including cervical mediastinoscopy (to exclude N2, N3 mediastinal lymph node metastases). The role of incomplete (palliative) resection is highly questionable, and therefore a complete *en bloc* excision is the aim of surgery. This usually includes:

- An appropiate pulmonary resection. This is generally a lobectomy, but on occasion a pneumonectomy may be necessary. A wedge excision of the upper lobe would be considered a compromise resection, but may be appropriate for selected patients with poor lung function. Mediastinal lymph nodes should be sampled/resected as for any lung cancer operation.

- Chest wall. All involved ribs, generally the entire first rib, and usually ribs 2 and 3.
- Vertebrae. Transverse processes may be removed *en bloc*. However, it is difficult to obtain a clear margin when resecting vertebral body, and long-term survival of patients with vertebral involvement is unusual. A multidisciplinary surgical approach (i.e. neurosurgeons and/or orthopedic surgeons in addition to thoracic surgeons) is advisable for tumors with significant involvement of the spine.
- Thoracic nerves up to the intervertebral foramen. The T1 root should be identified carefully (below the neck of the first rib), and may be divided with impunity. Division of C8 (in addition to T1) will result in considerable morbidity (poor hand function), and this must be balanced against the benefit of achieving a complete resection.
- Thoracic sympathetic chain and a portion of the stellate ganglion.
- Subclavian vessels. To achieve a complete resection, the involved subclavian vein may be resected *en bloc* and the ends suture-ligated. Invasion of the subclavian artery is a relative contraindication to resection. Technically part of the vessel may be resected, but vascular reconstruction or bypass may be necessary.

1. Approaches
- Posterolateral thoracotomy, using a long posterior incision up to the level of C7.
- Anterior approach (Dartevelle). The transclavicular approach requires thorough familiarity with the anatomy at the base of the neck. An L-shaped incision is made from the angle of the mandible to the sternal notch and extended horizontally under the clavicle to the deltopectoral groove. This approach provides better access to the anterior neurovascular structures at the thoracic inlet, but limited access to the vertebrae and lung hilum.
- Hemiclamshell or trap-door incisions, combining a partial median sternotomy with anterolateral fourth interspace and/or transverse cervical incisions.

2. Chest-wall reconstruction. Generally not required for posterior defects, as these are covered by the scapula. If the fourth rib is excised, the tip of the scapula should be excised to avoid this becoming trapped by the rib edge, or a prosthetic mesh should be utilized. Anterior defects usually require reconstruction.

Combined modality therapy	Only a few patients with well-localized disease and small tumors will benefit from radical surgical excision alone. Most patients receive combined therapy, as follows.

1. Preoperative radiation therapy. Radiotherapy doses range from 30 to 45 Gy and are usually given 4–6 weeks prior to surgical resection. Preoperative radiotherapy appears to improve resection rates from 10 to 25%, with minimal increased operative morbidity. Five-year survivals up to 45% are reported, if mediastinal nodes are negative. Incomplete resection, subclavian artery, vertebral body invasion (T4) and mediastinal lymph node metastases (N2, N3) are assocaited with poor long-term survival.

2. Postoperative radiation therapy. There is no established role for postoperative radiotherapy following complete resection of lung cancer. However, it is generally given for microscopic residual disease with the aim of reducing local recurrence.

3. Chemotherapy. Clinical trials are ongoing to define the role of systemic chemotherapy in this disease.

Further reading

Dartevelle PG, Chapelier AR, Macchiarini P. Anterior transcervical–thoracic approach for radical resection of lung tumors invading the thoracic inlet. *Journal of Thoracic and Cardiovascular Surgery,* 1993; **105:** 1025.

DeMeester TR, Albertucci M, Dawson PJ. Management of tumor adherent to the vertebral column. *Journal of Thoracic and Cardiovascular Surgery,* 1989; **97:** 373.

Detterbeck FC. Pancoast (superior sulcus) tumors. *Annals of Thoracic Surgery,* 1997; **63:** 1810.

Ginsberg RJ. Resection of superior sulcus tumors. *Chest Surgery Clinics of North America,* 1995; **5:** 315.

Komaki R, Mountain CF, Holbert JM. Superior sulcus tumors: treatment selection and results for 85 patients without metastasis (M0) at presentation. *International Journal of Radiation Oncology Biology and Physics,* 1990; **19:** 31.

Related topics of interest

PECTUS DEFORMITIES

Chris Compeau, Michael R. Johnston

A variety of congenital anterior chest-wall abnormalities have been described, ranging from deformity of the bony skeleton to absence of chest-wall structures. The etiology of these disorders is not known with certainty, although they are thought to arise as a result of abnormal (overgrowth or undergrowth) costal cartilage development. A positive family history of related chest-wall deformity is obtained in about one-third of patients, and a high incidence of chest-wall defects is seen in association with scoliosis and Marfan's syndrome. Surgical correction is generally indicated for cosmetic reasons.

Pectus excavatum

This deformity is characterized by depression of the sterum and lower costal cartilages, with sparing of the first and second ribs and manubrium. Rotation and asymmetry is common, and it is associated with scoliosis and a family history. Cardiopulmonary abnormalities are variable, but of questionable clinical significance. Patients may have reduced total lung capacity and/or reduced exercise tolerance. Specific physiological derangements are not usually identified. The timing of surgical correction is controversial. It should not be performed before 2 years of age. Repair before the infant starts school, or after the adolescent growth phase, is optimal.

Surgery
- Primary indication is cosmesis; physiologic indications are doubtful.
- Transverse (submammary) or vertical (midline) incision. Subperichondrial resection of involved costal cartilages. Wedge osteotomy of sterum with 10–15° overcorrection. The sternum is supported by wire sutures or a metal strut. Pectoral muscle is used to cover the sterum.
- Complications are rare. The most serious are pneumonthorax and wound infection.
- Recurrence rates are variable.

Pectus carinatum

An anterior protrusion deformity of the chest wall, referred to as a 'pigeon breast'. Upper condromanubrial deformity is common, and may be associated with rotational or excavatum defects. A family history of chest-wall deformity (25%) and scoliosis (13%) is common. The chondromanubrial defect is associated with congenital heart disease, but cardiopulmonary abnormalities are otherwise uncommon.

Surgery. Approaches are similar to those for an excavatum defect, involving a subperichondrial resection of deformed costal cartilages and sternal osteotomy.

Poland syndrome	The congenital absence of pectoralis major and minor muscles. Poland syndrome has an associated spectrum of chest-wall and breast deformities (hypoplasia, amastia) and also associated hand deformities, for example: hypoplasia (brachydactyly), fused digits (syndactyly) and claw deformity (ectromelia).

Surgery. Careful assessment of the extent of musculoskeletal involvement is essential. If an underlying sternal or costal cartilage deformity is demonstrated, subperichondrial resection with sternal osteotomy is required. Subsequent breast augmentation may be required. The absence of ribs may require chest-wall reconstruction with split rib grafts, mesh and latissimus dorsi muscle flaps.

Sternal defects Failure of fusion of the ventral thoracic wall may be classified as follows:

1. Cleft sternum. The cleft may be complete or incomplete, with the underlying midline visceral structures intact. Primary repair is performed in the newborn period.

2. Thoracic ectopia cordis. The cleft sternum is associated with other cardiac anomalies; the heart is uncovered and external to the thorax. Few neonates have been treated successfully.

3. Thoracoabdominal ectopia cordis (Cantrell's pentalogy). Comprises a cleft lower sternum, an anterior diaphragmatic defect, the absence of parietal pericardium, an omphalocele and cardiac anomalies (often tetralogy of Fallot). Salvage is possible with an aggressive surgical approach.

Further reading

Ravitch MM. *Congenital Deformities of the Chest Wall and their Operative Correction.* Philadelphia: WB Saunders, 1977.

Shamberger RC, Hendren WH. Congenital deformities. In: Pearson FG, Deslauriers J, Ginsberg RJ, Hiebert CA, McKneally MF, Urschel HC, eds. *Thoracic Surgery.* New York: Churchill Livingstone, 1995; 1189.

PERFORATED ESOPHAGUS

Donna E. Maziak, F. Griff Pearson

Esophageal perforation continues to carry a high mortality because of the difficulty in diagnosis and management. About 60% of perforations involve the thoracic esophagus, 24% the cervical esophagus and 16% the abdominal esophagus. The causes of esophageal perforation are quite diverse, but by far the most common is iatrogenic.

Etiology

1. Iatrogenic (57%)
- Instrumentation of the upper aerodigestive tract, including esophagogastroscopy (rigid and flexible), esophageal dilatation, nasogastric intubation, sclerotherapy, endotracheal intubation, rigid bronchoscopy.
- Operative, including pulmonary resection, mediastinoscopy, anti-reflux surgery, spinal surgery.

2. Traumatic (24%)
- Blunt and penetrating trauma.
- Foreign body.
- Caustic injury.

3. Spontaneous (19%)
- Postemetic (Boerhaave's syndrome).
- Thoracic tumors.

Clinical presentation

Specific symptoms and signs vary according to the level and duration of perforation, and whether complications have developed.

1. Cervical esophagus. Neck pain, dysphagia and odynophagia. Subcutaneous emphysema may be demonstrated on examination, and severe pain on neck movement or palpation is typical.

2. Thoracic and abdominal esophagus. Substernal or epigastric pain, radiating to the back. Dysphagia is variable. Examination may reveal subcutaneous air in the neck, peritonitis, dullness and reduced air entry, commonly at the left lung base.

3. General. Patients generally appear systemically ill, with tachycardia, hypotension, pyrexia, tachypnoea. Rapid clinical deterioration is usual.

Diagnosis

A high index of suspicion will often lead to the diagnosis of esophageal perforation. The diagnosis may be suspected on CXR or by the finding of air in the mediastinum, soft tissues of the neck, or in the abdomen. An associated pleural effusion (usually left sided) or an air–fluid level may be seen. Definitive diagnosis requires a contrast study, which will localize the level of perforation and demonstrate associated foregut pathology. Water-soluble contrast is given initially. If a perforation is not demonstrated, dilute barium should always be used. Esophagogastroscopy (using flexible fiberoptic instrumentation) is performed under general anesthesia, just prior to surgery to identify the perforation site (if possible) and assess esophagus at, as well as below, the perforation. Specifically, the presence of tumor or evidence of a distal obstruction will impact on surgical management.

Management

The principles of treatment are to stop ongoing soilage, eliminate infection, restore continuity of the esophagus, correct any underlying disorder and maintain nutrition. Immediate surgery offers the best chance of survival. Specific approaches depend on the anatomic location of the perforation, the time between perforation and diagnosis, and associated disorders.

1. General
- Preoperatively. Resuscitation with intravenous fluids, antibiotics (initially broad spectrum with oral anerobic coverage), oxygen therapy, drainage of associated pleural effusions (chest tube).
- Postoperatively. Nutritional support and culture-directed antibiotic therapy.

2. Cervical esophageal perforation. Prompt exploration using a left neck incision is performed, with extensive drainage of the retropharyngeal space and upper mediastinum. There is little place for nonoperative management of a cervical perforation. A primary repair (reinforced) is performed if possible (rare). A contrast study should be performed at 5–7 days postoperatively, and if no leakage demonstrated, oral intake can be resumed.

3. Thoracic esophageal perforation. Esophagogastroscopy following the induction of general anesthesia may help plan the operative approach. Upper and mid-thoracic esophageal perforations are best approached using a right thoracotomy, and lower perforations using a left thoracotomy. The entire length of the mucosal perforation should be visualized by dissecting the overlying muscle layers. Ideally a primary repair of healthy mucosa is performed (over a bougie), buttressed by local tissues (i.e. pleura, pericardium, intercostal muscle). Any mediastinal and pleural collections are drained extensively. Chest tubes are placed adjacent to the repair (in anticipation of postoperative leakage), and the lung is re-expanded. A mini-laparotomy is performed to place a feeding jejunostomy. The repaired perforation may be 'excluded' from salivary secretions by positioning a nasogastric tube in the esophagus with the tip just proximal to the repair (generally ineffective) or by creating a 'spit fistula' in the neck (cervical esophagostomy). Although very effective, this requires subsequent closure of the fistula. The repair can be protected from refluxed gastric or duodenal contents by ligation (or stapling) of the esophagogastric junction or placement of a decompressive gastrostomy tube (high on the lesser curvature in the event that stomach may be used for a later reconstruction). The decision to exclude the esophagus was recommended previously for the management of late (>24 hours) perforations. However, it is now reserved for patients who have failed primary repair of the perforation, or in whom primary repair is not feasible because of profound sepsis or severe mediastinitis. In the absence of distal obstruction, T-tube drainage (a controlled esophago-pleuro-cutaneous fistula) and wide drainage of the posterior mediastinum may be used when a primary repair cannot be performed. Benign esophageal disorders are corrected at the time of repair (i.e. myotomy for achalasia). Esophageal resection (with immediate or delayed reconstruction) should be considered early, especially in the presence of extensive esophageal injury, or for resectable tumors, where satisfactory palliation and quality of life may be achieved.

4. Abdominal esophageal perforation. Similar principles apply to the management of abdominal esophageal perforations. A laparotomy is performed, and all peritoneal collections are evacuated. It is not usually necessary to drain the peritoneum. Primary esophageal repairs are reinforced with either gastric fundus or omentum.

5. Nonoperative management. Selected patients, who meet strict criteria, who refuse surgery, or who have a prohibitive operative risk, may be considered for nonoperative management. However, full supportive therapy is required, including intravenous fluids, antibiotics, intervention and drainage of pleural or abdominal collections, and nutritional support. The criteria for nonoperative intervention, in patients otherwise suitable for surgery, are as follows.

- The leak is contained within the mediastinum.
- Contrast esophagram confirms free drainage back into the esophagus.
- There are minimal symptoms.
- There are no signs of clinical sepsis.

All patients treated in this manner should be followed very carefully, and evidence of local or systemic sepsis should prompt immediate surgical intervention. The stenting of perforated esophageal tumors and chest-tube drainage of the pleural space has been successfully used for patients with inoperable esophageal cancers.

Results
Current mortality rates for patients operated on within 24 hours of esophageal perforation are 13%; and 55% for patients in whom surgery is delayed. Mortality is also influenced by age, general medical condition, associated esophageal disease, etiology and location (thoracic >abdominal >cervical) of the perforation. Postoperative morbidity remains high (>40%) in most series.

Further reading

Brauer RB, Liebermann-Meffert D, Stein HJ, Bartels H, Siewert JR. Boerhaave's syndrome: analysis of the literature and report of 18 new cases. *Diseases of the Esophagus*, 1997; **10:** 64.

Cameron JL, Kieffer RF, Hendrix TR. Selective nonoperative management of contained intrathoracic esophageal disruptions. *Annals of Thoracic Surgery*, 1979; **27:** 404.

Ferguson MK. Management of perforated esophageal cancer. *Diseases of the Esophagus*, 1997; **10:** 90.

Iannottoni MD, Vlessis AA, Whyte RI, Orringer MB. Functional outcome after surgical treatment of esophageal perforation. *Annals of Thoracic Surgery*, 1997; **64:** 1606.

Jones WG, Ginsberg RJ. Esophageal perforation: a continuous challenge. *Annals of Thoracic Surgery*, 1992; **53:** 534.

Orringer MB, Sterling MC. Esophagectomy for esophageal disruption. *Annals of Thoracic Surgery*, 1991; **49:** 35.

Whyte RI, Iannettoni MD, Orringer MB. Intrathoracic esophageal perforation: the merit of primary repair. *Journal of Thoracic and Cardiovascular Surgery*, 1995; **109:** 140.

Related topics of interest

PERICARDIAL EFFUSION

Chris Compeau, Michael R. Johnston

The pericardium comprises a tough fibrous outer layer, and an inner serosal layer that is reflected onto the epicardium (visceral pericardium) and adventitia of the great vessels. Pericardial fluid is produced by the serosal layer, and represents the dynamic process of production (ultrafiltration) and resorption. Normally 15–50 ml of pericardial fluid are present within the pericardial space. Impairment of pericardial function by intrapericardial fluid accumulation (i.e. effusion), or reduced compliance (i.e. constrictive pericarditis), may alter cardiovascular hemodynamics, requiring prompt diagnosis and treatment.

Pathophysiology and etiology

A pericardial effusion results when the net rate of fluid production exceeds resorption. Rapid fluid accumulation increases the pressure gradient across the myocardium, compressing the right atrium and ventricle. This initially produces an elevated central venous pressure without significant hemodynamic consequences. With further fluid accumulation, diastolic filling is reduced, resulting in a decrease in stroke volume, cardiac tamponade and cardiogenic shock.

1. Malignancy (75%). Metastases from breast and lung carcinomas are the most common causes. Direct invasion may occur from mediastinal tumors (i.e. lymphoma, thymoma, mesothelioma, teratoma, angiosarcoma).

2. Benign (25%). May be a result of acute pericarditis (viral, idiopathic, bacterial, mycobaterial), traumatic, following myocardial infarction, post radiation therapy (may occur months to years later), uremic, aortic dissection, ruptured aneurysm or anticoagulants.

Clinical presentation

Depends on the rate of fluid accumulation rather than the volume of pericardial fluid. May be asymptomatic initially. A high index of suspicion should be maintained in patients with a history of acute viral pericarditis (3–7 days prodrome, fever, malaise, myalgia, chest pain, dyspnea, cough), malignancy, renal failure and an enlarged cardiac silhouette on CXR.

Acute tamponade. Beck's triad of distended neck veins, muffled heart sounds and hypotension. Patients with hemodynamically significant pericardial effusions can increase cardiac output only by increasing heart rate. A friction rub and pulsus paradoxicus may be present.

Diagnosis

- Chest X-ray. Enlarged cardiac silhouette.
- EKG. Low QRS voltage, ST changes, electrical alternans (acute pericarditis: ST elevation, no Q waves, T-wave inversion).

- Echocardiography. Pericardial fluid, hemodynamic compromise, compression of RV/RA, paradoxical septal motion, systolic collapse of RV/RA.

Management

1. *No hemodynamic compromise*
- Treat underlying condition: viral, analgesics or NSAIDs; post radiotherapy, steroids; uremic, increase frequency of dialysis.
- Diagnostic pericardiocentesis (guided by echocardiography).

2. *Impending or acute tamponade*
- Volume expansion, even with an elevated CVP to increase diastolic filling and right atrial pressure above intrapericardial pressure.
- Pericardiocentesis. For diagnosis; as definitive or interim therapy. May be performed under local anesthesia using a parasternal or subxiphoid route. The needle may be guided by echocardiography, radiology or by attachment to a praecordial EKG lead (deflects if contact is made with the myocardium). A drainage catheter may be positioned using the Seldinger technique. If malignant cells are demonstrated cytologically, or if the effusion recurs, sclerosis may be performed.

3. *Surgical decompression of pericardium.* Surgery is indicated for clotted blood, trauma, purulent pericarditis, loculated effusions, recurrent effusions, or for diagnostic biopsy of the pericardium. A subxiphoid pericardial window can be performed under local anesthesia through a small upper midline incision. A small portion of pericardium is removed for diagnosis, fluid is evacuated and cultured, and a small right-angle chest tube is placed in pericardium. A left anterior thoracotomy, or VATS, approach requires general anesthesia. A window is made in the pericardium by resecting the portion anterior to the phrenic nerve. Fluid then drains into the left pleural space. This is a good approach when the patient also has symptomatic left pleural effusion. Pericardiectomy is reserved for concomitant constrictive pericarditis. It is best approached through median sternotomy with resection of all pericardium anterior to the phrenic nerves.

Further reading

Girardi LN, Ginsberg RJ, Burt ME. Pericardiocentesis and intrapericardial sclerosis: effective therapy for malignant pericardial effusions. *Annals of Thoracic Surgery*, 1997; **64:** 1422.

Hancock EW. Neoplastic pericardial disease. *Cardiology Clinic*, 1990; **8:** 673.

Press OW, Livingstone R. Management of malignant pericardial effusion and tamponade. *Journal of the American Medical Association*, 1987; **257:** 1088.

Related topics of interest

Pleural effusion (p. 197)
Trauma (p. 265)

PLEURAL EFFUSION

Chris Compeau, Michael R. Johnston

Pleural effusions remain a common clinical problem, and thoracic surgeons are frequently called upon to help investigate and manage this problem. This requires an understanding of the pathophysiology of the pleural space, the limitations of noninvasive imaging modalities and a knowledge of current surgical approaches to the pleura, especially VATS.

Pathophysiology

The pleural space is a dynamic environment where 5–10 l of fluid are produced and reabsorbed daily. Under normal cirumstances only 5–20 ml of pleural fluid is present at any one time. Pleural homeostatsis may be altered by a variely of pathologic processes which act to increase fluid production and/or decrease fluid resorption.

1. Transudates
- Congestive heart failure.
- Hepatic failure.
- Renal failure.

2. Exudates
- Infections (bacterial, tuberculous, fungal, parasitic, viral).
- Collagen vascular disease (rheumatoid, lupus, Wegener's, ctc.).
- Malignancy (mesothelioma, lung cancer, metastases, lymphoma, etc.).
- Pulmonary embolus.
- Abdominal disease (pancreatitis, subphrenic abscess, etc.).
- Drug induced.
- Hemothorax.
- Chylothorax.
- Miscellaneous (esophageal perforation, sarcoidosis, radiation therapy, iatrogenic, postoperative, Meigs' syndrome, etc.).
- Idiopathic.

Malignant pleural effusions

Several thoracic and distant malignancies produce pleural effusions. Common mechanisms described are impaired lymphatic drainage (i.e. pleural implants, lymphatic metastases), increased pleural oncotic pressure (i.e. hypoalbumenemia, pleural implants, etc.), increased capillary permeability (i.e. infection, pleural implants), and increased venous pressure (i.e. superior vena cava obstruction (SVCO), malignant ascites). Malignant effusions are often bloody and the majority (i.e. 60–80%) will yield positive cytology on thoracentesis. As prognosis is poor (3–11 months median survival), any treatment provided is palliative.

Relative incidence
- *Males.* lung > lymphoma > GI tract > GU tract > mesothelioma.
- *Females.* breast > ovary > lung > lymphoma > GI tract > GU tract.

Diagnosis

1. Clinical presentation. A small effusion may be asymptomatic. Shortness of breath, cough and chest discomfort are the usual respiratory symptoms associated with an increasing effusion. Large effusions or those under tension may cause lethargy and a low output syndrome. Additional symptoms and signs may relate to the underlying disease process. Physical examination reveals diminished breath sounds and dullness to percussion consistent with pleural fluid.

2. Radiology. A fluid level, or meniscus, is characteristic. Blunting of the costo-diaphragmatic angle is an early radiologic sign, but already indicates the accumulation of several hundred milliliters (usually >400 ml) of fluid. A lateral decubitus film is helpful to confirm the presence of free-flowing (vs. loculated) pleural fluid. CT scanning is now widely used to image pleural effusions (particularly when loculated), and to assess underlying lung tissue and associated intrathoracic pathology. This imaging modality, along with ultrasound, is also useful to localize fluid prior to thoracentesis and for planning biopsy or surgery.

3. Thoracentesis. Aspiration of pleural fluid should be considered early to establish a diagnosis. Although this is a relatively straightforward procedure, it should be performed with care and using a sterile technique.

(a) Nature of fluid. Bloody effusions occur most commonly with malignancy, after a traumatic tap and with pulmonary embolus or tuberculosis. Milky fluid suggests a chylothorax. Pus is diagnostic of an empyema.
(b) Microbiology for culture and sensitivity.
(c) Cytology.
(d) Biochemistry. Many parameters have been proposed for diagnosis of a pleural effusion. However, the following are the most useful in current clinical practice.
- Total protein. Defines an exudate (>3 g/dl) vs. a transudate (<3 g/dl). The ratio of pleural protein/serum protein is <0.5 in a transudate, and >0.5 in an exudate.
- LDH. Ratio of pleural LDH/serum LDH >0.6 suggests an exudate.
- Glucose. Low (<60 mg/dl) suggests malignancy, tuberculosis, parapneumonic effusion or rheumatoid effusion.

- pH. A parapneumonic effusion with low pH (<7.0) suggests progression to empyema.
- Amylase. Elevated in pancreatitis, esophageal perforation, malignant effusions.
- Triglycerides. High levels (>110 mg/dl) are diagnostic of a chylothorax.
- Pleural complement/ rheumatoid factor/ antinuclear antibody are often elevated in collagen vascular diseases.

4. Pleural biopsy. Percutaneous biopsy alone yields a diagnosis of malignancy in 40–70% of cases. This may be increased with multiple biopsies (at the risk of pneumothorax, however), or when combined with pleural fluid cytology. This technique may be helpful to diagnose amyloidosis or tuberculosis, when cytology is not informative. Thoracoscopy, especially if guided by CT findings, should improve the diagnostic yield to over 95%. The recent development of minimally invasive approaches (i.e. VATS) has expanded the potential for early diagnosis considerably. A bronchoscopy should also be performed to exclude endobronchial disease. Occasionally rigid (open tube) pleuroscopy or even mini-thoracotomy are required to obtain an adequate pleural biopsy.

Management

In general, most transudative effusions should resolve following treatment of the underlying cause. Selective exudates (i.e. collagen vascular disease, drug induced) will also resolve with appropriate therapy of the underlying condition. Establishment of a precise diagnosis, evacuation of all pleural fluid and ensuring that the underlying lung will re-expand (CT scanning to assess pleural thickness, bronchoscopy to exclude an endobronchial obstruction and a trial of thoracentesis) are essential to the successful palliative management of malignant pleural effusions.

Pleurodesis. Following chest-tube drainage, or at thoracoscopy, insertion of various agents intrapleurally will promote pleural synthesis. For example sclerosants (i.e. talc, tetracycline) produce a chemical pleuritis, adhesions, and obliteration of the pleural space. Tetracycline was recently discontinued in North America, but is still available in the UK. It is inexpensive, may be administered through a chest tube, and is reported to be 40–80% successful. The major disadvantage is fever and pleuritic pain, although the latter may be controlled by concurrent intrapleural administration of local anesthetics. There has therefore been renewed interest in use of talc (5–10 g as a slurry or poudrage at thoracoscopy). Previous concerns about the long-term use of talc (particularly malignancy) were related to its preparation with asbestos. As talc preparation today is asbestos-free, and with a life-expectancy of less than 1 year predicted for most patients requiring palliative pleurodesis, talc continues to be used widely, with success rates approximating 60–80%.

Cytostatic agents (i.e. *C. parvum*, interleukin-2, cisplatin, 5-fluorouracil) are presumed to reduce pleural tumor volume. Success rates vary considerably; potential systemic toxicity, and cost have limited the use of many agents in routine clinical practice.

Most studies to evaluate the optimal agent for pleurodesis are retrospective and uncontrolled. A few prospective studies are reported, but are based on relatively few patients, heterogenous etiology of effusions, short follow-up and the lack of defined end-points (particularly related to symptoms and quality of life). They are further limited by the short life-expectancy of such patients.

Management of a malignant effusion/ trapped lung

Patients with malignant pleural effusions often have tumor in the lung parenchyma or visceral pleura which prevents full re-expansion of the lung. This condition presents a therapeutic challenge to the surgeon. In such cases evacuation of pleural fluid may improve symptoms, even if the lung does not re-expand fully. As failure to expand means that pleurodesis will fail, the following treatment options exist.

1. Pleuroperitoneal shunt. Patient-activated subcutaneous pump to drain pleural fluid into the peritoneum.

2. Tenckhoff catheter. External silastic drainage catheter. Patients may aspirate pleural fluid as required.

3. Decortication. A surgical procedure to remove the constricting visceral pleural peel in an attempt to expand the underlying compressed lung. Excessive morbidity and mortality generally outweighs palliative benefit. May be useful for selected 'good risk' patients only.

Further reading

Belani CP, Pajeau TS, Bennett CL. Treating malignant pleural effusions cost consciously. *Chest*, 1998; **113 (Suppl.):** 78S.

Moores DW. Management of the malignant pleural effusion. *Chest Surgery Clinics of North America*, 1994; **4:** 243.

Patz EF. Malignant pleural effusions: recent advances and ambulatory sclerotherapy. *Chest*, 1998; **113 (Suppl.):** 74S.

Robinson RD, Fullerton DA, Albert JD, Sorensen J, Johnston MR. Use of pleural Tenchoff catheter to palliate malignant pleural effusion. *Annals of Thoracic Surgery*, 1994; **57:** 286.

Ruckdeschel JC. Management of malignant pleural effusions. *Seminars in Oncology*, 1995; **22:** 58.

Related topics of interest

PNEUMOTHORAX

Chris Compeau, Michael R. Johnston

A pneumothorax is simply defined as air in the pleural space. This results in secondary lung collapse, and may progress to hemodynamic and respiratory instability. Treatment of a pneumothorax is dicated by the underlying cause and the severity of patient symptoms.

Classification and etiology

1. *Spontaneous*
   (a) Primary – ruptured apical bleb. A bleb is defined as a subpleural collection of air contained within the visceral pleura. They are usually small (below 3 cm) and are located at the apex of the upper lobe or superior segment of the lower lobe. The etiology of blebs is not clear, although it is believed that they are a form of localized interstitial emphysema (periacinar, paraseptal).
   (b) Secondary – associated with:
   - Chronic obstructive lung disease. Usually secondary to rupture of a bulla, defined as an air-filled space located within the lung parenchyma. They result from alveolar-wall destruction associated with emphysema.
   - Cystic fibrosis.
   - Infection. Cavitating pulmonary infections (bacterial, mycotic, parasitic) and tuberculosis are particularly prone to develop pneumothorax.
   - Acquired immune deficiency syndrome. Usually secondary to *Pneumocystis carinii* pneumonia, but may occur with Kaposi's sarcoma, mycobacterial and cytomegalovirus infection. Bilateral, recurrent pneumothoraces, with persistent bronchopleural fistulae, are typical.
   - Tumors. Rupture of ischemic primary or metastatic lung tumors (lung carcinomas, lymphomas, sarcomas) may occasionally result in pneumothorax. May also develop during chemotherapy.
   - Catamenial. Associated with menstruation (usually within 48–72 hours), usually right-sided and recurrent. The pathogenesis is unclear, but focal endometrial implants on the pleura, and several other mechanisms, are proposed.
   - Miscellaneous. Marfan's syndrome, Ehlers–Danlos syndrome, histiocytosis X, eosinophilic granuloma, sarcoidosis, lymphangiomyomatosis, and other connective tissue/autoimmune diseases.

2. *Traumatic*
   (a) Iatrogenic – lung biopsy, central line insertion, mechanical ventilation (barotrauma).
   (b) Noniatrogenic – penetrating or blunt chest trauma (dis-

ruption of tracheobronchial tree, pulmonary parenchyma, esophageal perforation).

Clinical presentation

1. Symptoms. Related to the degree of pulmonary collapse and underlying lung function. May be asymptomatic. Symptoms (dyspnoea, chest pain, occasional nonproductive cough) may occur during rest or exercise. Primary spontaneous pneumothorax typically occurs in tall young male patients. In a patient over 50 years of age with a history of chronic lung disease, sudden respiratory distress (hypoxia, hypercarbia, acidosis) should suggest the development of a secondary pneumothorax. Even a small pneumothorax may not be tolerated because of limited pulmonary function.

2. Signs. Physical examination may reveal few signs with a small pneumothorax. Diminished breath sounds and hyperresonance are otherwise typical.

3. Radiology. An erect PA and lateral X-ray will confirm the diagnosis. A small pneumothorax will be accentuated by an expiratory film. A CT is useful to differentiate pulmonary cysts and bullae in the presence of subcutaneous emphysema, when lung markings may not be easily seen on standard films. It may also be used to quantitate the degree of pneumothorax, overcoming the limitations of many formulae based on standard radiography.

Complications

1. Persistent air leak. Most air leaks will seal within 48 hours, with good pleural drainage (i.e. adequate chest tube, suction), and re-expansion of the underlying lung. Persistence is more likely with secondary pneumothorax, and implies the presence of a bronchopleural fistua.

2. Recurrence. Risk after the first episode is estimated to be up to 20% within 2 years. The rate of recurrence increases to over 50% after a second pneumothorax (first recurrence), and subsequently.

3. Bilateral. Occur in fewer than 10% of patients sequentially; and in 1% of patients simultaneously.

4. Tension pneumothorax. Develops in 2–3% of patients, when alveolar air enters the pleural space but is not resorbed, usually because of a one-way valve mechanism. Intrapleural pressure increases and exceeds atmospheric pressure throughout expiration, resulting in respiratory failure (altered lung mechanics, mediastinal shift, reduced ventilation, increased shunt, decreased tissue oxygenation) and cardiovascular collapse (tachycardia, reduced stroke volume).

5. *Hemothorax.* A rare complication (<5%) resulting from tearing of a vascular adhesion between the lung and chest wall.

6. *Pneumomediastinum.* Secondary to dissection of air along bronchovascular structures.

Treatment

1. *Observation.* Used if a patient is asymptomatic and the pneumothorax is small (<20%), with no evidence of radiologic progression. Absorption of air is estimated at 1.25% of the volume of hemithorax/24 hours. Hospitalization is recommended initially, but a resorbing pneumothorax may be followed as an outpatient. The disadvantage of this approach is the potential for developing complications (i.e. tension pneumothorax), and the need for prolonged observation. Medical therapy of underlying lung disease should also be initiated.

2. *Aspiration.* Simple aspiration of air manually, using a 16 gauge angiocath, a three-way stopcock and a 60 ml syringe (or suction bottle) is estimated to be successful in only 20–50% of patients.

3. *Chest-tube drainage.* This remains the most effective technique provided a sufficiently large tube (no less than 28 F) is used. This is connected to an underwater seal and suction (–20 cmH$_2$O) to ensure complete re-expansion of the underlying lung. A persistent air leak should be managed by surgery, the timing of which depends on the etiology. If the patient is high-risk for anesthesia (or refuses surgery) conversion to underwater seal drainage alone, or use of a one-way chest-drainage system (flutter-valve, with bag) for use as an outpatient, may be successful, provided the lung remains expanded.

4. *Pleurodesis.* The aim of this technique is to obliterate the pleural space by creating an intense inflammatory reaction between the visceral and parietal pleura using various agents, most often tetracycline or talc. Most surgeons do not favor the routine use of this approach, especially for young patients who may require thoracotomy later in life. Recurrence rates are also high (20–40%) compared with surgery.

5. *Surgery.* The indications for surgery are as follows.
- Prolonged air leak.
- Failure of the underlying lung to re-expand.
- Occupational hazard (i.e. airline pilots, divers).
- Tension pneumothorax.
- Single large bulla.
- Bilateral pneumothoraces.
- Hemopneumothorax.
- Recurrent pneumothoraces.

The aim of surgery is to resect underlying blebs or bullae, and to obliterate the pleural space to prevent recurrence. This may be achieved by thoracotomy (axillary, muscle-sparing) or using minimally invasive techniques (VATS). Rarely is a median sternotomy necessary. The preferred approach to bilateral disease is simultaneous staged VATS. It is important to also perform a bronchoscopy to exclude an endobronchial lesion that may prevent re-expansion of the underlying lung. Surgical resection of blebs or bullae is readily achieved using mechanical stapling devices. Coagulation of bullae or blebs using electrocautery, laser and argon beam (especially thoracoscopically) is reported to control air leaks and bleeding, but recurrence rates up to 25% are reported. Pleural synthesis is achieved by pleurectomy or mechanical pleural abrasion. Recurrence rates are less than 1%.

Primary spontaneous pneumomediastinum

- Uncommon, usually seen after physical effort (males).
- Results from tracking of interstitial air (from alveolar rupture along peribronchial and perivascular spaces to reach the mediastinum and neck.
- Benign clinically, although appearances may be alarming.
- Occasionally dyspnoea and cough may be present. A continuous murmur over the apex of the heart (Hamman sign) and subcutaneous emphysema may be present.
- Treatment is by observation alone. Techniques for surgical decompression are described, but are rarely necessary.
- It is essential to exclude an associated condition requiring further treatment, including pneumothorax, tracheobronchial injury, esophageal perforation or perforated abdominal viscus (resulting in pneumoperitomeum).

Further reading

Deslauriers J, Beaulieu M, Despres JP. Transaxillary thoracotomy for the treatment of spontaneous pneumothorax. *Annals of Thoracic Surgery*, 1980; **30:** 35.

Hazelrigg SR, Landreneau RJ, Mack MJ. Thoracoscopic stapled resection for spontaneous pneumothorax. *Journal of Thoracic and Cardiovascular Surgery*, 1993; **105:** 389.

Paape K, Fry WA. Spontaneous pneumothorax. *Chest Surgery Clinics of North America*, 1994; **4:** 517.

Related topics of interest

Bronchopleural fistula (p. 29)
Chest tubes (p. 42)
Hemothorax (p. 132)
Trauma (p. 265)

POSTOPERATIVE MANAGEMENT AND COMPLICATIONS

Ziv Gamliel, Alan G. Casson

Successful postoperative management of thoracic surgical patients requires careful attention to detail. Every effort should be made to recognize potential complications early, as prompt management will reduce postoperative morbidity and mortality. The first section summarizes the general features of postoperative management, and the second reviews the spectrum of postoperative complications most often encountered in thoracic surgical practice.

General postoperative management

Monitoring

Most postoperative cardiorespiratory complications occur during the first 2–4 days, and therefore initial monitoring is best achieved in a specialized unit (i.e. high-dependency unit) that is capable of providing information on the following parameters:

- Continuous cardiac rhythm.
- Arterial blood pressure.
- Central venous pressure.
- Arterial oxygen saturation.
- Fluid status: daily weights, urine output.
- Chest-tube patency and drainage.

Formal admission to an intensive care unit is generally reserved for patients requiring ventilation, and specialized hemodynamic monitoring.

Pain control

Post-thoracotomy pain is often severe and results in a reduction in tidal volume, avoidance of coughing resulting in atelectasis and impaired clearance of secretions. Significant progress in pain control has been made in recent years, especially with the epidural infusion of narcotics or local anesthetics. Other pain-control strategies include patient-controlled analgesia (PCA) with parenteral narcotics, or NSAIDs (oral or rectal). However, attentive bedside monitoring of a patient's analgesic needs and judicous administration of parenteral narcotics by experienced nursing personnel still provides the optimum combination of pain control and overall nursing care.

Pulmonary therapy

- Adequate analgesia to obtain a reasonable comfort level without causing sedation.
- Routine use of chest physiotherapy, preferrably by dedicated therapists.

- Encouragement of independent coughing and deep breathing.
- Early and frequent ambulation.
- Oxygen therapy, titrated to maintain adequate O_2 saturation (usually 90% or greater) and prompt discontinuance of supplemental oxygen when no longer medically indicated. This discourages oxygen dependance and promotes free ambulation.
- For patients with an inadequate cough or copious secretions, airway suctioning may be required. This can be accomplished by bedside nasotracheal suction catheter insertion, flexible fiberoptic bronchoscopy or on occasion, tracheostomy.
- Ventilation of selected patients only (i.e. following prolonged anesthesia, after massive transfusions or fluid administration and to achieve maximal lung re-expansion after decortication).

Fluid administration

Pulmonary surgery is not typically associated with large fluid shifts, but following intraoperative lung manipulation, excessive fluid administration may easily result in pulmonary edema. Patients undergoing pneumonectomy are particularly prone to fluid overload and right heart failure because of a marked increase in pulmonary vascular resistance. Their fluid status should be monitored carefully. Daily weights, monitoring of CVP and urine output reflects general fluid status. Patients undergoing esophageal resection generally require larger volumes of fluids (often >3 l/day) in keeping with the extensive dissection and obligate third space fluid loss.

Postoperative complications

Postoperative morbidity and mortality

In current clinical practice, 30-day postoperative mortality following elective lobectomy is approximately 2–3%, and for pneumonectomy is approximately 6–8% (right > left). Minor morbidity following elective lobectomy is approximately 40–50% and is approximately 35–75% for elective pneumonectomy. Major complications occur in about 10% of cases only. Extended pulmonary resections (i.e. including chest wall, pericardium), and bronchoplastic procedures (i.e. sleeve resection) are associated with an increased risk of mortality (up to 20%). Major causes of death following pulmonary surgery are respiratory failure, pneumonia, bronchopleural fistula/empyema, myocardial infarction and pulmonary embolus. Mortality following elective esophagectomy is approximately 5%. However, morbidity rates approximate 40%, of which half will be due to major complications. Morbidity and mortality rates should be reviewed by individual surgeons, and in thoracic surgical units within the framework of quality control (North America) or audit (UK).

Respiratory complications Respiratory failure is the main cause of postoperative mortality in thoracic surgery, and is estimated to occur in up to 2% of patients, with a 50–100% mortality. Careful preoperative assessment will identify patients at increased risk, who require additional management measures.

1. Aspiration. Pulmonary aspiration (massive or silent) occurs in up to 25% of patients undergoing general anesthesia. Additional predisposing factors, related to thoracic surgical procedures involving the upper aerodigestive tract, include prolonged intubation (nasogastric, endotracheal, tracheostomy, feeding tubes, T-tubes), esophageal dysfunction resulting in impaired clearance or regurgitation, and recurrent laryngeal nerve palsy (i.e. following pneumonectomy, cervical esophagogastrostomy). A high index of suspicion should be maintained in patients who develop respiratory failure within the first 4 postoperative days (even in the absence of a witnessed event), with prompt management aimed at respiratory and circulatory support. The use of steroids and antibiotics is controversial. If a paralyzed vocal cord (abducted) is diagnosed, early augmentation (glycerol, temporary; Teflon, permanent) should be considered, although late recovery (or compensation) is often seen.

2. Pneumonia. Aspiration, airway colonization, impaired host defenses (i.e. reduced mucociliary clearance, decreased alveolar macrophage function), and reduced cough resulting in atelectasis, may all contribute to the development of postoperative pneumonia. Culture-directed antibiotic therapy, vigorous physiotherapy and respiratory support, remains the mainstay of treatment.

3. Bronchopleural fistula/empyema. See 'Bronchopleural fistula', p. 29 and 'Empyema', p. 75.

4. Lobar gangrene. Torsion of the remaining lobe(s) after lobectomy results in vascular and bronchial obstruction, pulmonary infarction and lobar gangrene. Patients typically present with pyrexia, hemoptysis, relatively normal blood gases (lack of lobar perfusion) and serial X-ray findings of increased parenchymal opacification. Although CT and bronchoscopy may be helpful for the diagnosis, a high index of suspicion should be maintained, and the patient returned to surgery. Detorsion may salvage a viable lobe, which should be fixed to prevent recurrence; otherwise if ischemic injury is severe, lobectomy will be required.

Cardiac complications

1. Cardiac herniation. A rare complication of lung resection requiring intrapericardial dissection, arising in the immediate postoperative period, comprising sudden onset of hypotension, tachycardia and cyanosis. Although characteristic radiologic signs are described, a high index of clinical suspicion should prompt re-exploration and detorsion. Primary closure of the pericardium is recommended. However, enlarging the pericardial defect to allow free herniation without inflow obstruction is an acceptable maneuver when large portions of the pericardium have been resected particularly on the left side.

2. Cardiac failure. Frequently presents as hypotension or oliguria. The first consideration is to optimize intravascular volume, and measurement of CVP or pulmonary wedge pressure is helpful. Cardiac output may be enhanced by afterload reduction (nitroglycerine or nitroprusside) or by increasing myocardial contractility with inotropic drugs (dopamine, dobutamine). Correction of hypoxia, acidosis and electrolyte abnormalities is essential. Right heart failure following pneumonectomy is particularly difficult to treat and has a high mortality rate.

3. Myocardial infarction. Usually occurs on the second or third postoperative day. Chest pain may be difficult to evaluate after thoracotomy and cardiac enzymes difficult to interpret in the immediate postoperative period. Serial EKGs may be more helpful. Myocardial ischemia or infarction should be managed in the usual manner pharmacologically (i.e. nitrates, calcium channel blockers, etc.), with antiarrhythmic therapy and with inotropic support/afterload reduction based on monitoring hemodynamic status.

4. Cardiac dysrhythmias. Cardiac dysrhythmias (especially atrial fibrillation) occur with a peak incidence at 48 hours. They are detected in up to 15% of patients undergoing lobectomy, and in up to 40% of patients undergoing pneumonectomy. The precise etiology of cardiac dysrhythmias following thoracotomy is unclear, but general factors (i.e. electrolytes, acid–base status, oxygen saturation) should be assessed and corrected as necessary. The pharmacologic therapy of established dysrhythmias requires a precise diagnosis, and the urgency of therapy depends on the degree of hemodynamic compromise. Several prospective studies have failed to show a benefit from prophylactic digitalization.

Postpneumonectomy pulmonary edema

May present 24–72 hours after pneumonectomy (right > left), especially in patients who receive large volumes of intravenous fluid perioperatively. Mortality rates are high (>50%), and it is believed that the pathophysiology is related to altered vascular permeability. The precise etiology is unclear although rapid hyperinflation of the remaining lung with major mediastinal shift has been implicated. Patients experience increasing dyspnoea, initially with a clear CXR, which later shows radiographic signs of pulmonary edema. Differential diagnoses include pulmonary embolus, congestive heart failure, aspiration and pneumonia. Prompt diuresis, and fluid restriction, may resolve very mild cases, but often progression is rapid and mechanical ventilation is required.

Renal complications

Urine output less than 0.5 ml/kg/hour requires evaluation. Oliguria (<400 ml/day) suggests prerenal or renal failure, whereas anuria (<100 ml/day) suggests urinary tract obstruction, renal vascular obstruction or acute cortical necrosis. Management includes careful attention to fluid and electrolyte balance, with dialysis for uncontrolled electrolyte abnormalities, fluid overload unresponsive to diuretic therapy, acidosis, and to remove nephrotoxic agents.

Esophageal anastomotic leaks

Esophagogastric, -colonic or -jejunal anastomotic leaks can occur at any stage postoperatively, although most present (clinically or radiologically) between days 3 and 7 postoperatively. The clinical spectrum of presentation ranges from an asymptomatic, localized anastomotic leak, detected incidentally on a routine postoperative contrast study, to necrosis of the conduit with massive leakage, mediastinal and pleural sepsis. Prompt diagnosis of a suspected leak should be made using radiologic contrast studies: initially, water-soluble contrast, and if negative, dilute barium. Prognosis and management, depends on the anatomic location (i.e. intrathoracic or cervical), the extent of local sepsis and tissue viability. Most leaks in the neck respond to local drainage, whereas a necrotic conduit will require excision, defunctioning of the foregut (i.e. spit fistula, feeding jejunostomy) and later reconstruction. Associated mediastinal and pleural abscesses should be drained; antibiotics are used to control systemic sepsis.

Further reading

Deslauriers J, Ginsberg RJ, Piantadosi S, Fournier B. Prospective assessment of 30-day operative morbidity for surgical resections in lung cancer. *Chest*, 1994; **106 (Suppl.):** 329S.
Grillo HC, Shepard JO, Mathisen DJ, Kanarek DJ. Postpneumonectomy syndrome: diagnosis, management and results. *Annals of Thoracic Surgery*, 1992; **54:** 638.

Ritchie AJ, Danton M, Gibbons JR. Prophylactic digitalisation in pulmonary surgery. *Thorax*, 1992; **47:** 41.

Von Knorring J, Lepantalo M, Lindgren L, Lindfors O. Cardiac arrhythmias and myocardial ischemia after thoracotomy for lung cancer. *Annals of Thoracic Surgery*, 1992; **53:** 642.

Waller DA, Gebitekin C, Saunders MR. Walker DR. Noncardiogenic pulmonary edema complicating lung resection. *Annals of Thoracic Surgery*, 1993; **55:** 140.

Yano T, Yokoyama H, Fukuyama Y, Takai E, Mizutani K, Ichinose Y. The current status of postoperative complications and risk factors after a pulmonary resection for primary lung cancer: a multivariate analysis. *European Journal of Cardiothoracic Surgery*, 1997; **11:** 445.

Related topics of interest

PREOPERATIVE ASSESSMENT FOR THORACIC SURGERY

Fang Gao, Ziv Gamliel

A successful outcome in general thoracic surgery depends not only on technical expertise and judgement in the operating room, but also on careful patient selection. The aims of preoperative evaluation are to confirm the diagnosis, to determine the need for surgical intervention, to assess co-morbid disease, and to identify patients at increased risk for postoperative complications. As the majority of postoperative complications following general thoracic surgery are cardiopulmonary, this section will focus on preoperative cardiopulmonary assessment. It is important to recognize that surgery is now performed on an aging population, where associated cardiopulmonary disease is prevalent, and that with improved anesthesia (analgesia), increasing numbers of patients with relatively poor pulmonary function may now be considered suitable for pulmonary resection.

Predictors of postoperative morbidity and mortality (most significant)

- Cardiovascular disease.
- Pulmonary disease.
- General medical condition
  Age >70 years,
  Nutritional status (i.e. weight loss >10%),
  Associated chronic disease (i.e. diabetes),
  Immunosuppression.
- Tumor stage/extent of resection.
- Psychosocial factors (i.e. attitude toward illness, or surgery).

Cardiovascular assessment

The risk of postoperative myocardial infarction following general anesthesia is estimated at <0.1%. The risk increases for patients with:

- A previous infarct within 3 months of surgery.
- Unstable angina pectoris.
- Congestive heart failure (uncontrolled).
- Hypertension.
- Valvular disease.
- Dysrhythmias and conduction defects.

An overall estimation of cardiac risk may be estimated using the Goldman cardiac risk index, which classifies patients by a score derived from a multivariate analysis of selected preoperative risk factors (i.e. recent myocardial infarct, congestive heart failure, aortic stenosis, EKG alterations, arterial blood gases, age, type of surgery).

In addition to a full history, physical examination, CXR and EKG, the following preoperative cardiac investigations may be required for high-risk patients.

- Exercise stress test.
- Exercise thallium imaging. May identify reversible myocardial ischemia requiring further investigation with coronary angiography and potential revascularization prior to thoracotomy. Patients with a negative scan (or a fixed defect) are at low risk for a perioperative cardiac event.
- Coronary angiography. Should be considered in patients with unstable or poorly controlled symptoms and in patients with objective evidence of coronary ischemia.

Pulmonary assessment

Pulmonary complications following thoracic surgery are the most common cause of postoperative morbidity and mortality. Most patients are current or ex-smokers, with some degree of coexisting pulmonary disease, whose respiratory mechanics are further impared by a posterolateral thoracotomy or an upper abdominal incision.

1. History and examination. The degree of dyspnoea generally does not correlate well with objective studies of pulmonary function. A careful history of activity level and limitations is an important adjunct to pulmonary function testing (and often more revealing). The ability to climb two flights of stairs and converse normally (without dyspnea) suggests adequate pulmonary function for pneumonectomy (and general fitness for surgery). In patients with productive cough, sputum should be sent (preoperatively) for bacteriologic culture and antibiotic sensitivity. Examination should detect cyanosis, stridor, pattern and rate of breathing, added chest sounds, stridor and venous engorgment suggestive of superior vena caval obstruction, etc.

2. Radiography. The plain CXR and CT scan are helpful in evaluating the anatomic extent of pulmonary disease.

3. Pulmonary function studies. Objective preoperative evaluation of pulmonary function is useful to identify high-risk patients undergoing thoracic surgery, and to predict postoperative quality of life. Many studies are available, with various degrees of sophistication. It should be remembered that each individual test (in isolation) has limitations, and often several are required to develop a composite picture of pulmonary function. As there is no absolute criterion to contraindicate thoracotomy (and pulmonary resection), often considerable clinical judgement must be used. See 'Pulmonary function studies', p. 215 for further information.

Preoperative preparation

Selected patients identified by preoperative studies as high risk may respond to the following measures, to improve cardiopulmonary function to a point where surgical risk is minimized.

This may be achieved in a supervised, structured pulmonary rehabilitation program, which includes a graded and measured exercise program for 3–4 weeks preoperatively.

- Cessation of smoking. A reduction in carboxyhemoglobin is seen after 2–3 days, and a reduction in airway secretions and reactivity is seen after 2–4 weeks.
- Treatment of bronchospasm with bronchodilators and steroids.
- Reduction of pulmonary secretions by chest physiotherapy, adequate hydration, prophylactic antibiotics.
- Correction of anemia.
- Rehydration and nutritional support.
- Correction of specific disorders (i.e. congestive heart failure, cardiac dysrhythmias).

Further reading

Goldman L, Caldera DL, Nussbaum SR, Southwick FS, Krogstad D, Murray B, Burke DS, O'Malley TA, Goroll AH, Caplan CH, Nolan J, Carabello B, Slater E. Multifactorial index of cardiac risk in noncardiac surgical procedures. *New England Journal of Medicine*, 1977; **297**: 845.

Mangano DT, Goldman L. Preoperative assessment of patients with known or suspected coronary disease. *New England Journal of Medicine*, 1995; **333**: 1750.

Markos J, Mullan BP, Hillman DR, Musk AW, Antico VF, Lovegrove FT, Carter MJ, Finucane KE. Preoperative assessment as a predictor of mortality and morbidity after lung resection. *American Review of Respiratory Disease*, 1989; **39**: 902.

Prause G, Offner A, Ratzenhofer-Komenda B, Vicenzi M, Smolle J, Smolle-Juttner F. Comparison of two preoperative indices to predict perioperative mortality in non-cardiac thoracic surgery. *European Journal of Cardiothoracic Surgery*, 1997; **11**: 670.

Zeldin RA, Math B. Assessing cardiac risk in patients who undergo noncardiac surgical procedures. *Canadian Journal of Surgery*, 1984; **27**: 402.

Related topics of interest

Anesthesia for thoracic surgery (p. 8)
Postoperative management and complications (p. 206)
Pulmonary function studies (p. 215)

PULMONARY FUNCTION STUDIES

Ziv Gamliel

Pulmonary complications following thoracic surgery are the most common cause of postoperative morbidity and mortality. Chronic pulmonary disease is prevalent in the population of patients undergoing thoracic surgery, many of whom are smokers or ex-smokers. Furthermore, respiratory mechanics are impaired by thoracotomy or upper abdominal incisions. One of the aims of preoperative evaluation is to predict patients at increased risk for postoperative pulmonary complications, and objective assessment of pulmonary function remains an essential component of overall assessment. It should be recognized that many tests are available, and that each in isolation has limitations. Therefore, several tests are often required to develop a composite picture of pulmonary function.

Summary of pulmonary physiology

The purpose of the respiratory system is to deliver oxygen to, and remove carbon dioxide from, the tissues. The coordination and regulation of this process is complex. Conducting airways extend from the nasopharynx to the terminal bronchioles, where convection is the mode of gas transport. Beyond this level, diffusion occurs, transporting gas to the acinus (i.e. respiratory bronchioles, alveolar ducts, sacs and alveoli) where gas exchange occurs. Gas exchange occurs across the thin air/blood barrier, comprising the alveolar epithelium (type I and II pneumocytes), capillary epithelium and a fused basement membrane. The balance between hydrostatic and oncotic pressures results in fluid migration from the air spaces to the interstitium and vascular space. The lung and chest wall are elastic structures with inherent recoil and different mechanical properties, resulting in complex pressure–volume relationships.

Lung volumes may be divided into several compartments (*Figure 1*). The following are most useful:

1. *Tidal volume.* The volume of air during tidal breathing.

2. *Total lung capacity.* The total volume of air within the lungs at maximal inspiration.

3. *Vital capacity (forced vital capacity).* The volume of air expired, from maximal inspiration to full expiration.

4. *Residual volume.* The volume of air remaining after maximal expiration, which can not be exhaled. This is determined by respiratory muscle strength, chest-wall compliance and airway closure. With increasing age, airway closure occurs at higher volumes (independent of muscle strength), and residual volume rises from approximately 20% (age 20 years) to 40% (age 70 years).

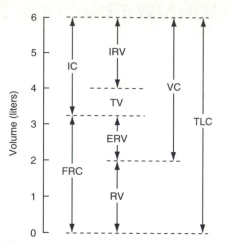

Figure 1. The volumes of the lung. ERV, expiratory reserve volume; FRC, functional residual capacity; IC, inspiratory capacity; IRV, inspiratory reserve volume; RV, residual volume; TLC, total lung capacity; TV, tidal volume; VC, vital capacity.

5. Functional residual volume (capacity). The volume remaining after expiration during tidal breathing. This represents the volume at which the inward recoil of the lung balances the outward recoil of the chest wall. It is reduced in obesity and pregnancy, and increased with chronic obstructive lung disease.

Maximum emptying of the lungs is only possible with forced expiratory airflow. Flows between 25 and 75% of total forced expiratory flow (or maximum midexpiratory flow) are largely effort independent, but offer no practical advantage to measurements of forced expiratory volume in 1 second (FEV_1) or its ratio with forced vital capacity (FEV_1/FVC).

Measurement of pulmonary function

Expiratory airflow and lung volumes are measured by a combination of spirometry (volume/time or flow/volume) and more specialized tests (i.e. helium dilution, constant-volume body plethysmography, flow transducers). Normal values are based upon sex, age and height. It should be appreciated that considerable variation may exist between laboratories, and that equipment should be calibrated carefully on a regular basis.

Spirometry

1. Forced expiratory volume in 1 second. FEV_1 may be expressed as an absolute value (normally >2 l) or as a percentage of predicted. This is the most widely used predictor of postoperative pulmonary morbidity, which increases significantly in patients with a postoperative FEV_1 of 800 ml or less.

2. Ratio of FEV_1 to forced vital capacity. A normal ratio of FEV_1/FVC is approximately 70–80%. In obstructive lung disease, FEV_1 is reduced, but lung volumes are increased. The ratio is therefore reduced. In restrictive disease, both FEV_1 and FVC are reduced, maintaining a normal ratio.

3. Flow–volume curves. The shape of the flow–volume loop is dependent on the functional properties of the airways, lung volumes and recoil, and characteristic patterns will be found in restrictive disease, obstructive disease and with upper airway obstruction. Quantitative measurements of lung volume with respect to time can also be made from the inspiratory or expiratory curves.

Gas transfer tests

Carbon monoxide diffusing capacity (D_LCO) measures the uptake of carbon monoxide, to reflect the integrity of the air–blood interface. A value of <30% predicted represents high risk for major pulmonary resection.

Arterial blood gases may also be used to evaluate gas transfer and ventilation.

$PaCO_2$ provides the most useful information as it reflects adequacy of alveolar ventilation, and minimal alterations indicate severe dysfunction of gas exchange.

Exercise testing

Measurement of exercise capacity evaluates the combined performance of the cardiac and respiratory systems. Oxygen desaturation with exercise mandates further testing of cardio-respiratory function. Maximal oxygen uptake (VO_2max) is the most sophisticated preoperative predictor of outcome, but a lack of standardization between laboratories has limited its widespread use. It is used to identify surgical candidates who might otherwise be denied thoracotomy on the basis of borderline spirometry. In general, values <20 ml/kg/min are predictive of increased postoperative morbidity; values <10 ml/kg/min are prohibitive of major pulmonary resection.

Quantitative perfusion/ventilation scanning

Radionuclide lung perfusion/ventilation scanning estimates the contribution of each lung, or region, to global lung function. It is a relatively simple, noninvasive test, that has largely replaced bronchospirometry and lateral position testing. Quantitation of lung perfusion may be used, in combination with spirometry, to accurately predict pulmonary function (i.e. FEV_1, D_LCO, vital capacity) after resection. This is particularly useful in patients with borderline spirometry, where for pneumonectomy:

Postop FEV_1 = preop $FEV_1 \times$ % function of remaining lung.

Similar calculations can be performed to predict lung function after lobectomy, based on regional function of the lobe to be resected.

Six-minute walk	This is an inexpensive, easily performed and reproducible test of cardiorespiratory reserve. It has been used most extensively in patients with chronic obstructive lung disease, but recent evidence supports its use in the preoperative evaluation of thoracic surgery patients. Patients are instructed to walk on a predetermined course as far and as fast as they can. Distances over 1000 feet (305 m) has been correlated with an uncomplicated postoperative recovery.
Stair climb	For years thoracic surgeons have advocated walking patients upstairs as an informal means of assessing exercise tolerance. A few authors have attempted to formalize this into a submaximal test with measures of workload and VO_2max. Others have used breathlessness or a decrease in O_2 saturation after ascending two flights of stairs as indicators of risk.
Clinical applications of pulmonary function studies	1. *Preoperative evaluation*. See 'Preoperative assessment for thoracic surgery', p. 212.

2. *Diagnosis of functional pulmonary disorders*
(a) Obstructive ventilatory disorders
- Chronic obstructive pulmonary disease (generic).
- Chronic bronchitis.
- Emphysema.
- Asthma.
- Cystic fibrosis.
- Bronchiolitis obliterans.
(b) Restrictive ventilatory disorders
- Fibrosing alveolitis.
- Interstitial pneumonitis/ fibrosis.
- Sarcoidosis.
- Chest-wall deformities.

Further reading

Crapo RO. Pulmonary function testing. *New England Journal of Medicine*, 1994; **331:** 25.
Gass GD, Olsen GN. Preoperative pulmonary function testing to predict postoperative morbidity and mortality. *Chest*, 1986; **89:** 127.
Olsen GN, Bolton JW, Weiman DS, Hornung CA. Stair climbing as an exercise test to predict postoperative complications of lung resection. *Chest*, 1991; **99:** 587.

Related topics of interest

PULMONARY METASTASES

Sean Grondin, Michael R. Johnston

Historically, the presence of pulmonary metastases was thought to represent advanced disease in which surgical intervention was contraindicated. However, recent published data suggest that surgical resection results in a signficiant survival advantage in selected patients.

Pathology

The lung is the most common site of metastasis for all malignancies. These most often develop following hematogenous spread, although it is increasingly recognized that the biology of the primary tumor and host resistance ('seed and soil') may be responsible for patterns of metastasis, growth rates, etc. The systemic nature of metastasis implies that the majority of patients will potentially have multiple sites of metastases (or micrometastases), although autopsy studies report 'isolated' pulmonary metastases in up to one-third of patients. For most sarcomas, the lung is the first site of metastatic involvement.

Diagnosis

As most metastases are peripheral lesions, few patients are symptomatic. Diagnosis is typically made on follow-up CXR after resection of a primary tumor. The optimal frequency of follow-up is not known, although in current clinical practice this is carried out 3-monthly. CT scanning is then used to evaluate suspicious lesions in selected patients. Although CT scanning can detect smaller pulmonary metastases than plain X-ray, no data exist as to whether survival is improved by earlier detection. This must also be balanced against radiation exposure and cost.

Principles of resecting pulmonary metastases

Few curative treatment options exist for patients with metastatic solid tumors. Resecting lung metastases is appropiate if:

- The primary tumor has been successfully controlled.
- Metastatic disease is limited to the lung, with no other extrathoracic disease demonstrated.
- All metastases in the lung must be resected. Resections should utilize lung-sparing techniques as much as possible since multiple reoperations are often necessary to keep the lung clear of metastases.
- Operative risk is acceptable, with adequate cardiopulmonary function.
- If metastases recur following resection (growth of micrometastases), reoperation is indicated provided the patient still meets surgical prerequisites.

Surgical techniques

Various approaches have been described. The lung is carefully palpated and all suspicious lesions are resected. Typically twice as many lesions are found at surgery as were seen on preoperative imaging studies, but some will be benign nodules. Most metastases are present subpleurally, and may be resected by wedge excision with a margin of normal lung, using a surgical stapler. This achieves maximal preservation of lung parenchyma. The adequacy of resection margins must be assessed by the surgeon. Anatomic segmentectomy or lobectomy may be necessary for central lesions. Selected patients may benefit from more extended resections, including pneumonectomy, *en bloc* resection of chest wall or other thoracic structures, provided a complete excision is achieved.

1. Median sternotomy. The preferred approach for initial exploration of both thoracic cavities. Bilateral disease may be resected at one procedure, although exposure of the posterior hilae and left lower lobe may be difficult. Less patient discomfort.

2. Posterolateral thoracotomy. Utilized with large posterior tumors, especially in elderly patients. Performed as staged procedures for bilateral disease.

3. Bilateral anterior thoracotomies (clamshell incision). Gives good exposure to both lungs but has higher morbidity than median sternotomy.

4. Video-assisted thoracoscopic surgery (VATS). Gives minimal morbidity, good visualization and useful for diagnosis, especially if associated pleural lesions. However, current technology limits the ability to evaluate fully the lung parenchyma.

Prognostic factors

The following predictors of outcome may be used to identify patients who are most likely to benefit from resection of pulmonary metastases. In current clinical practice, no single factor has been found to exclude patients from resection. The relative importance of each factor also appears to depend on the tumor being evaluated.

- Resectability. The most constant single variable reflecting postoperative outcome.
- Length of disease-free interval (time between treatment of the primary tumor and diagnosis of metastasis). For most tumors studied, a disease-free interval greater than 12 months is associated with prolonged survival. May reflect tumor biology.
- Tumor-doubling time. Calculated using a mathematical formula based on radiologic measurement of tumor dimensions. For soft-tissue sarcomas, a tumor doubling time greater than 20 days was reported to be associated with prolonged survival. Associations for other tumors are less clear.

- Number of metastases on preoperative imaging and resected surgically. Improved outcome is seen with limited numbers of metastases (generally less than three to four, depending on tumor histology). In patients with renal cell carcinoma, melanoma and breast cancer, number of nodules does not appear to influence outcome.
- Tumor histology.
- Age, gender and primary tumor site, have generally not been found to influence post-thoracotomy survival.

Results

Surgical resection can be performed safely (minimum morbidity and mortality) for patients with a wide range of metastases. Most series report 5-year survival rates of 20–40%, with the following specific differences.

- Germ-cell tumors do best, melanoma worst (68% vs. 21% at 5 years).
- Survival with osteogenic sarcoma is better than with soft-tissue sarcoma (35% vs. 25% at 5 years). Of the soft-tissue sarcomas, malignant fibrous histiocytomas had the most favorable outcome.
- Epithelial tumors (carcinomas) generally have up to 37% survival at 5 years.

Further reading

Casson AG, Putnam JB, Natarajan G, Johnston DA, Mountain C, McMurtrey M, Roth JA. Efficacy of pulmonary metastasectomy for recurrent soft tissue sarcoma. *Journal of Surgical Oncology*, 1991; **47:** 1.

Gruenwald D, Spaggiari L, Girard P, Baldeyrou P, Filaire M, Dennewald G. Completion pneumonectomy for lung metastases: is it justified? *European Journal of Cardiothoracic Surgery*, 1997; **12:** 694.

McCormack PM, Ginsberg KB, Bains MS, Burt ME, Martini N, Rusch VW, Ginsberg RJ. Accuracy of lung imaging in metastases with imlications for the role of thoracoscopy. *Annals of Thoracic Surgery*, 1993; **56:** 863.

Putnam JB, Suell DM, Natarajan G, Roth JA. Extended resection of pulmonary metastases: is the risk justified? *Annals of Thoracic Surgery*, 1993; **55:** 1440.

Robert JH, Ambrogi V, Mermillod B, Dahabreh D, Goldstraw P. Factors influencing long-term survival after lung metastasectomy. *Annals of Thoracic Surgery*, 1997; **63:** 777.

Roth JA, Pass HI, Wesley MN, White D, Putnam JB, Seipp C. Comparison of median sternotomy and thoracotomy for resection of pulmonary metastases in patients with adult soft-tissue sarcomas. *Annals of Thoracic Surgery*, 1986; **42:** 134.

REOPERATION FOR FAILED ANTI-REFLUX SURGERY

Donna E. Maziak, F. Griff Pearson

The best results following anti-reflux surgery are obtained at the time of the initial procedure, and depend on the establishment of a precise diagnosis, careful patient selection and skilled operative intervention. However, a long-term failure rate of 10–20% is to be expected, even by experienced surgeons and regardless of the initial anti-reflux procedure performed. Reoperation for failed anti-reflux operations is often technically challenging, but with careful patient selection, satisfactory results may be achieved.

Causes of failure

1. Functional causes
- Failure of the fundoplication to prevent reflux.
- Failure of esophageal clearance, or an underlying motility disorder.
- Failure of both the fundoplication and esophageal clearance.
- Bile (or mixed) reflux.

2. Anatomic causes
- Inappropriate anti-reflux procedure for a primary motility disorder.
- Failure to recognize an anatomically short esophagus.
- Fundoplication too loose, too tight or too long.
- Disruption of the fundoplication or slipping of the wrap down onto the stomach below the esophagogastric junction (slipped Nissen).
- Hiatal hernia with migration of the fundoplication into the chest.
- Recurrent reflux with peptic stricture.
- Paraesophageal hernia.
- Inappropriate anti-reflux procedure for peptic ulcer disease.

Diagnosis

It is essential to review the operative notes and preoperative investigations from the initial procedure. Following a comprehensive history and physical examination, the following objective studies are performed to assess the foregut anatomy, and to define as precisely as possible, disordered esophagogastric physiology.

- A barium swallow.
- An esophagogastroscopy.
- Esophageal manometry.
- Ambulatory 24-hour pH studies.

Additional studies (i.e. radionuclide gastric clearance, ambulatory bile reflux studies, etc.) may also be indicated to further confirm the diagnosis.

Management

1. Medical. Patients are treated with medications similar to those given for primary reflux. Although some patients respond well to this approach, medical management is less successful when an anatomic cause of failure has been identified.

2. Dilatation. Patients with dysphagia, who are found to have a tight fundoplication, may benefit from gradual serial dilatation with Maloney or Savary dilators. Balloon dilation appears to be too disruptive and less effective in this situation.

3. Reoperation. Individual cases for reoperation should be selected with particular care, and the implications of further surgery explained in detail to the patient and relatives. Although no single procedure is applicable to all patients, optimal exposure of the foregut may be achieved using a thoracoabdominal approach, which is generally well tolerated.

If the underlying problem is a primary motility disorder, the fundoplication is taken down, and a myotomy performed with a partial (Belsey) fundoplication. If a disrupted wrap, a short esophagus or 'slipped Nissen' is found, the previous repair is taken down and reconstructed with a Collis gastroplasy and either a partial (Belsey) or total (Nissen) fundoplicaton, based on preoperative motility studies. If the patient has had multiple operations or a persistent undilatable distal esophageal stricture, esophageal resection with interposition of colon or jejunum should be considered For bile (or mixed) reflux, acid suppression and bile diversion by antrectomy and Roux-en-Y gastrojejunostomy may occasionally be required.

Further reading

Collard JM, Romagnoli R, Kestens PJ. Reoperation for unsatisfactory outcome after laparoscopic antireflux surgery. *Diseases of the Esophagus*, 1996; **9:** 56.

Ellis FH, Gibb SP. Vagotomy, antrectomy, and Roux-en-Y diversion for complex reoperative gastroesophageal reflux disease. *Annals of Surgery*, 1994; **220:** 536.

Skinner DB. Surgical management after failed antireflux operations. *World Journal of Surgery*, 1992; **16:** 359.

Stein HJ, Feussner H, Siewert JR. Failure of antireflux surgery: causes and management strategies. *American Journal of Surgery*, 1996; **171:** 36.

Related topics of interest

SMALL CELL LUNG CANCER

Sean Grondin, Michael R. Johnston

Small cell lung cancer (SCLC), sometimes referred to as oat cell cancer, represents approximately 20% of all lung cancers. It is considered separately because of its different biologic and clinico-pathologic features to non-small cell lung cancer (NSCLC).

Pathology

SCLC is an epithelial tumor capable of expressing neuro-endocrine amine precursor uptake and decarboxylase (APUD) markers, which can act as neurotransmitters, paracrine regulators or hormones. ACTH and ADH are the hormones most commonly overproduced. Histological examination shows very small (10–20 μm), round cells, with scanty cytoplasm and prominent, hyperchromatic nuclei. Mitoses are frequent, and there is characteristically absence of a defined architectural pattern. Mixed tumor histology (i.e. non-small cell or intermediate small cell components) is not uncommon. Examination by electron microscopy demonstrates neurosecretory granules. Immunohistochemistry may demonstrate the variable expression of markers, including neuron-specific enolase (NSE), chromogranin, bombesin, ACTH, calcitonin, vasoactive intestinal polypeptide (VIP), substance P and somatostatin. These are biologically aggressive tumors, with high rates of cell proliferation and characteristic patterns of molecular genetic alterations (i.e. *myc*, *Rb*, chromosome 3) compared with NSCLC.

Clinical presentation

These are clinically aggressive tumors, with a tendency to early dissemination. Metastatic disease may affect virtually any organ. Symptoms may be related to local tumor growth and invasion, regional lymph-node metastases, distant metastases or associated paraneoplastic syndromes. There is a strong association with cigarette smoking. Classic CXR imaging shows a large perihilar mass with bilateral bulky mediastinal lymphadenopathy. However, any radiologic pattern may be seen. A definitive tissue diagnosis is essential prior to therapy. Biopsy material may be difficult to interpret due to necrosis and 'crush artefact'.

Staging

1. Investigations
- History and physical examination.
- Routine hematology, liver function tests, alkaline phosphatase.
- Chest X-ray.
- CT of chest.
- CT or ultrasound of abdomen.
- Bone scan.

- CT or MRI of brain.
- Bone-marrow aspiration and biopsy is not performed routinely, except if peripheral blood analysis suggests marrow involvement.

2. *Staging*
- Limited disease. Originally defined as the area encompassed within a radiotherapy portal. Tumor confined to ipsilateral lung, hilar, mediastinal and supraclavicular lymph nodes. Ipsilateral malignant pleural effusion and SVCO are still considered limited disease.
- Extensive disease. Extrathoracic disease beyond the confines of limited disease. Includes contralateral lung and pericardial disease.
- Very limited small cell lung cancer. Suspected to be confined to the lung, and potentially suitable for surgical resection. Should be staged using the TNM system.

3. *Prognostic factors*
- Ambulatory performance status.
- Weight loss, serum albumin.
- Serum LDH.
- Limited vs. extensive disease

Management

Primarily treated with chemotherapy (systemic therapy); the most useful agents include cisplatin, vincristine, etoposide, cyclophosphamide and doxorubicin. Drug combinations have been shown to have better response rates than single-agent therapy. Appropriate treatment depends upon the stage of the disease, and assessment of prognostic factors. In general, about 90% of patients will have either a partial response (50% or greater decrease in size of measurable tumor) or a complete response (complete clinical or radiologic resolution of tumor) to therapy.

Extensive disease

- The majority of patients will have extensive disease at presentation.
- Combination chemotherapy is the preferred therapy.
- Complete response rate is about 30%.
- Five-year survival is <5%. Median survival is 8–12 months.
- Radiotherapy is used for palliation of symptoms such as brain metastasis, SVC syndrome or painful bone metstases.

Limited disease

- 30–50% of patients will present with limited disease.
- Approximately 50% of patients will have a complete response to therapy.
- Five-year survival may approach 20%. Median survival is 12–15 months.
- The most frequent site of first relaspe is within the thorax.

- Radiotherapy is superior to surgery in reducing the local failure rate and has become an integral adjuvant to chemotherapy in limited-stage SCLC.
- Combination chemotherapy plus concurrant thoracic irradiation has demonstrated a small but significiant survival benefit over sequential therapies. The role of hyperfractionated radiation therapy is controversial.
- Prophylactic cranial irradiaition (PCI) is recommended in patients with a complete response only. Although rates of CNS relapse are reduced, no survival benefit has been proven to date.

Role of surgery in SCLC
- Diagnosis and staging.
- Generally limited to resection of the rare SCLC that presents as a solitary pulmonary nodule.
- Very limited disease (T1, T2, N0 by TNM classficiation). Five-year survival rates of 60–70% may be seen when surgical resection is combined with chemotherapy. The sequence of chemotherapy and surgery does not appear to be critical. It is also not known whether this approach is superior to chemoradiotherapy.
- The role of induction chemotherapy followed by complete surgical resection of N1 or N2 tumors is also unclear, although a few studies have reported 5-year survival rates of up to 40% (especially for downstaged tumors).

Further reading

Ihde DC. Chemotherapy for small cell lung cancer. *New England Journal of Medicine*, 1992; **327:** 1434.

Murray N, Coy P, Pater J. Importance of timing for thoracic irradiation in the combined modality treatment of limited stage small cell lung cancer. *Journal of Clinical Oncology*, 1993; **11:** 336.

Pignon JP, Arriagada R, Ihde DC. A meta-analysis of thoracic radiotherapy for small cell lung cancer. *New England Journal of Medicine*, 1992; **327:** 1618.

Shepherd FA, Ginsberg RJ, Feld R. Surgical treatment for limited small cell lung cancer. *Journal of Thoracic Cardiovascular Surgery*, 1991; **101:** 385.

Shepherd FA, Ginsberg RJ, Haddad R. The importance of clinical staging in limited small cell lung cancer: a valuable system to separate prognostic subgroups. *Journal of Clinical Oncology*, 1993; **8:** 1592.

Wagner H. Radiation therapy in the management of limited small cell lung cancer: when, where and how much? *Chest*, 1998; **113 (Suppl.):** 92S.

Related topics of interest

SOLITARY PULMONARY NODULE

Michael R. Johnston

A solitary pulmonary nodule is defined as a discrete lung lesion 3 cm in diameter or less and completely surrounded by lung parenchyma. Thus lesions abutting pleura, diaphragm, mediastinum or within the lung hilum do not meet these criteria. The incidence varies with geographical location, age of cohort and local practice patterns regarding routine CXRs. Typically, these lesions are completely asymptomatic and come to medical attention when discovered incidentally on a CXR obtained for other reasons.

Etiology

1. *Inflammatory*
   - Granuloma from prior infection; most common are TB, histoplasmosis, coccidiodomycosis, blastomycosis.
   - 'Round pneumonia'.
   - Wegener's granulomatosis, sarcoidosis and rheumatoid nodules may be solitary but are usually multiple.

2. *Benign tumor*
   - Lung carcinoid.
   - Hamartoma.
   - Hemangioma.

3. *Malignant tumor*
   - Primary lung cancer.
   - Lung metastasis.

Significance

The major problem is to distinguish between a benign lesion (inflammatory or tumor) and an early stage, highly curable lung cancer. Lung cancer patients presenting with an asymptomatic solitary pulmonary nodule (clinical T1 N0) on a CXR have the best prognosis of any group with invasive lung cancer. Although lung cancer in general has only a 13% 5-year survival, T1 N0 M0 disease may have up to an 85–90% survival in bronchioloalveolar carcinoma (60–80% for other NSCLC histologies and about 25% with SCLC). Once nodal metastases develop, survival drops significantly.

Diagnostic imaging

A CXR from longer than 1 year before the most recent film showing the exact same lesion to be unchanged is strong evidence for benignity. A CXR or chest CT scan that shows 'popcorn' calcification (hamartoma) or concentric calcification (calcified granuloma) also imply a benign lesion. Spiculated lesions, those with scattered calcifications or with indistinct borders are highly suspicious for malignancy. CT scan determination of tissue density (in Houndsfield units) show benign lesions are generally more dense than cancers, but overlap is too great to be reliable. MRI offers no advantage over CT scan. PET scan appears to be more sensitive and specific than CT, with reported false negative rates less than 10%. More experience and wider availability are needed before strongly endorsing this technique.

Tissue diagnosis

- Sputum culture and skin tests may suggest a fungal or TB etiology but are not diagnostic.
- Bronchoscopy with bronchoalveolar lavage is low yield.
- Biopsy procedures: transbronchial biopsy is performed through a bronchoscope under fluoroscopic guidance. Small tissue fragments are obtained for histology. Successful biopsy is operator-dependent and becomes more difficult the more peripheral the lesion is located. Percutaneous needle biopsy is performed under fluoroscopic or CT guidance. Core needle biopsies can be obtained from lesions close to the chest wall, while more central lesions require fine needle aspiration (for cytologic diagnosis). All biopsy procedures have complications, namely bleeding, hemoptysis or pneumothorax. Tumor seeding is extremely rare. A biopsy showing malignancy is highly accurate but determination of the precise cell type is often problematic, especially with cytology specimens (~50% accurate). Biopsies showing benign tissue have a 15–30% incidence of false-negative results, meaning the nodule is really malignant even though a benign biopsy was obtained. Only if tissue gives a specific benign diagnosis (i.e. hamartoma) can it be believed with certainty. Tissue biopsies showing granulomas should be accepted as indicating a benign nodule with caution, since scar carcinomas are known to occur adjacent to old granulomatous lesions, especially when secondary to TB.

  Excisional biopsy can be performed by either open techniques (thoracotomy) or VATS – both give a definitive diagnosis. The nodule is removed totally with a margin (at least 2 cm) of normal lung tissue. VATS technique is appropriate if the nodule is close to the pleural surface. Needle localization methods and intraoperative ultrasound are under investigation as means of identifying lesions deep within lung tissue. Following excision, the nodule is immediately sent for frozen section analysis. If lung cancer is diagnosed, an open, definitive resection is then performed (usually lobectomy and lymph node dissection or sampling).

Treatment strategy

A new nodule in a middle-aged or older smoker is a primary lung cancer until proven otherwise. The chance of a solitary pulmonary nodule being lung cancer in this group is about the same as the patient's age. Choices of management include:

- Needle biopsy.
- Transbronchial biopsy.

- Excisional biopsy.
- Observation.

In individuals at low risk of cancer, poor operative risk patients, or those with nodules showing a benign appearance, observation with repeat CT scans at 3-monthly intervals is appropriate. Controversy exists as to whether the length of follow-up should be 1 or 2 years. Any growth of the lesion suggests malignancy and excision should be strongly considered. High cancer risk patients should have a CT scan to ensure that the lesion is solitary, and then offered surgical resection. Needle or transbronchial biopsy techniques are reserved for patients who are prohibitive operative risks or those who are reluctant to undergo surgery without a definitive diagnosis. In the future, PET scanning may obviate the need for biopsy procedures. Patients with a positive scan would go directly to surgical resection while the negative scan patients would be followed on a 3-monthly interval with CT to assess potential interval growth.

Further reading

Lillington GA, Caskey CI. Evaluation and management of solitary and multiple pulmonary nodules. *Clinics in Chest Medicine*, 1993; **14:** 111.

Naidich DP, Garay SM. Radiographic evaluation of focal lung disease. *Clinics in Chest Medicine*, 1991; **12:** 77.

Related topics

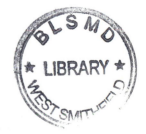

STENTS: AIRWAY

Shaf Keshafjee, Hani K. Najm

The purpose of a tracheobronchial stent is to maintain patency through a stricture or narrowing that is not amenable to resection and reconstruction. Tracheobronchical stents are used for benign and malignant strictures and can be left in place for extended periods. Silastic stents are placed using a variety of bronchoscopic techniques. Expandable wire stents have recently been introduced and can be successfully placed either bronchoscopically or by the interventional radiologist under fluoroscopic control.

Indications

- To maintain the patency of a malignant airway obstruction:
    Following removal of endobronchial tumor.
    For extrinsic compression from a tumor mass.
    For a stenotic airway following radiation therapy.
- Tracheoesophageal fistula (malignant).
- Benign tracheobronchial stenoses such as:
    Post tracheal resection.
    Post sleeve lobectomy.
    Prolonged intubation.
    Burn injuries.
    Nonresectable strictures.
    Post lung transplant.

Types

The silastic (silicone rubber) stent and the expandable wire stents are available in various diameters, lengths and configurations. Typically the silastic stent has a side-arm off the main channel that is brought out through a tracheostome to anchor the tube in the trachea (Montgomery T-tube). The main channel may also be bifurcated to accommodate obstructions at the carina (Y or T-Y configurations) or may be short and flanged for bronchial applications. The wire stents are available either with a thin synthetic covering or bare. They are preloaded in an applicator catheter which simplifies insertion.

Choice of stent and technique for insertion

The silastic stents require placement in the operating room under anesthesia. A rigid bronchoscope is inserted and the distance between the vocal cords and the obstruction noted. Strictures are dilated and malignant obstructions resected with biopsy forceps or the Nd:YAG laser. The silastic tube is inserted perorally or through a tracheal stoma with the T-arm extending out through the stoma. These tubes can be repositioned, removed or replaced with relative ease but sometimes develop occlusions from inspissated secretions.

The metal stents may be placed fluoroscopically, but if tumor resection or stricture dilation is necessary, bronchoscopy is still required. These stents are thin walled and well suited for bronchial obstructions and, if necessary, multiple stents can be placed. However, once in place they generally can not be repositioned or removed. Tumor may grow rapidly through the interstities of an uncovered stent or around either end. Their major limitation is probably their cost compared with the silastic tubes.

Results

Both stents work well for benign airway obstruction, although there is less long-term experience with the metal stents. Silastic stents can often become obstructed with dried secretions. Maintaining high humidity in the inspired air usually alleviates this problem. For malignant lesions stents provide reasonable palliation, although survival depends on the stage of disease.

Causes of failure

- Anatomic obstruction.
- Dried secretions.
- Aspiration.
- Progression of disease.

Complications

- Stent migration, possible obstruction of lobar orifice.
- Obstruction with secretions or tumor.
- Tracheoesophageal fistula.
- Tracheoinominate artery fistula.

Further reading

Cooper JD, Pearson FG, Patterson GA. Use of silicone stents in the management of airway problems. *Annals of Thoracic Surgery*, 1989; **47:** 371.

Dumon JF. A dedicated tracheobronchial stent. *Chest*, 1990; **97:** 328.

Gaissert H, Grillo HC, Mathisen DJ, Wain JC. Temporary and permanent restoration of airway continuity with the tracheal T-tube. *Journal of Thoracic and Cardiovascular Surgery*, 1994; **107:** 600.

Hramiec JE, Haasler GB. Tracheal wire stent complications in malacia: implications of position and design. *Annals of Thoracic Surgery*, 1997; **63:** 209.

Landa L. The tracheal T-tube. In: Grillo HC, Eschapasse H, eds. *International Trends in General Thoracic Surgery*. Philadelphia: WB Saunders, 1987; 124.

Rousseau H, Dahan M, Lauque D. Self-expandable prostheses in the tracheobronchial tree. *Radiology*, 1993; **188:** 199.

Related topics of interest

SUPERIOR VENA CAVA SYNDROME

Sean Grondin, Michael R. Johnston

The superior vena cava is located in the upper right medistinum, originating from the junction of the right and left brachiocephalic veins (behind the right first costal cartilage), and terminating in the right atrium (right third intercostal space). It drains venous blood fron the upper thorax, both upper limbs, and the head and neck. It is a large-diameter, thin-walled structure partially encircled by medistinal lymph nodes. Compression of this vessel by tumor or nodes leads to obstruction of venous flow, resulting in clinical and radiologic signs referred to as the superior vena caval obstruction (SVCO) syndrome. SVCO is usually a sign of advanced malignancy and surgical intervention, other than for diagnosis, is rarely indicated.

Etiology

The spectrum of disorders associated with SVCO has changed dramatically. Previously, benign causes (i.e. aortic aneurysm, tuberculous, syphilitic or fungal mediastinitis, idiopathic fibrosing mediastinitis) predominated.

Malignant thoracic disease accounts for the majority of cases today, predominantly cancers of the lung (70–80%). SVCO develops in approximatley 10% of patients with small cell lung cancer and in 3% of patients with non-small cell tumors. This may be explained by the more central location, and high incidence of nodal metastases, seen in small cell lung cancers. Other malignant causes include lymphoma (5–15%), mediastinal tumors (i.e. germ-cell tumors, thymic malignancy), metastases and rarely tumor embolus or angiosarcoma.

Benign diseases such as fibrosing medistinitis, substernal goiter and aneurysms of the great vessels are responsible from approximately 5% of cases.

Iatrogenic causes (i.e. thrombosis secondary to transvenous pacemakers or central venous lines), account for about 5% of cases. Associated thrombosis is estimated to occur in up to 50% of patients with malignant or benign SVCO.

Clinical presentation

SVCO generally develops insidiously, although sudden deterioration may occur (i.e. following acute thrombotic occlusion).

1. Symptoms. Dyspnoea (50%), cough (30%), facial or arm swelling (20%). Uncommon symptoms include chest pain, syncope, headache and confusion.

2. Signs. Edema and a prominent venous pattern of the head, neck, upper trunk and arms is found in over half of all patients; with cyanosis and plethora (20%), papilledema, Horner's syndrome and vocal cord paresis seen less frequently.

Diagnosis

- Chest X-ray may identify an anterior mediastinal mass.
- CT scan of the chest with intravenous contrast will show the level at which the SVC is obstructed, the extent of mediastinal disease and venous collaterals.

- MRI is useful in further defining mediastinal vascular anatomy.
- Venography to demonstrate the site of obstruction, the presence of intravascular thrombus and patterns of collateral vessels. Radionuclide scintigraphy is being used with increasing frequency, but does not allow accurate assessment of vascular anatomy.
- Serum markers β-HCG or α-fetoprotein if a germ-cell tumor is suspected.
- A histologic diagnosis is essential for definitive therapy. Commonly used procedures include: percutaneous needle biopsy, bronchoscopy, mediastinoscopy, mediastinotomy, VATS, or rarely, thoracotomy. In modern practice, such diagnostic studies are not associated with particularly increased morbidity.

Management

Previously considered a medical emergency, SVCO was treated somewhat empirically. The recognition of a changing etiology, that invasive diagnostic procedures can be performed safely, and the need to establish a tissue diagnosis prior to definitive therapy have recently influenced approaches to the management of SVCO. The goal of therapy is generally palliation of symptoms.

1. Medical. Nonspecific measures include elevation of the head, oxygen, diuretics and salt restriction. Intravascular volume should be maintained, however, to minimize risk of thormbosis. Steriods may be of benefit for patients with associated laryngeal edema or brain metastases. Anticoagulants are used when associated venous thrombosis is demonstrated, although a definitive advantage is not proven. Few studies have evaluated the role of thrombolytic therapy.

2. Radiotherapy. This remains the mainstay of treatment for thoracic malignancy. However, dose, fractionation and field size remain controversial.

3. Chemotherapy. This may be used alone when SVCO results from lymphoma or small cell lung cancer, or increasingly in combination with radiotherapy. A response is usually seen within 1 week of starting treatment.

4. Interventional radiology. Intravascular stents are being used with increased frequency (and success) to palliate SVCO resulting from benign and malignant disease.

5. Surgery. Surgical bypass is generally reserved for patients with benign disease, and for highly selected patients with malignancy, in whom long-term survival may occur. Several techniques are described, and venous autografts appear to have improved patency rates. Resection (and vascular reconstruction) is indicated for localized tumor involvement.

Further reading

Ahmann FR. A reassessment of the clinical implications of the superior vena caval syndrome. *Journal of Clinical Oncology*, 1984; **2:** 961.

Callejas MA, Rami R, Catalan M. Mediastinoscopy as an emergency diagnostic procedure in superior vena cava syndrome. *Scandinavian Journal of Thoracic and Cardiovascular Surgery*, 1991; **25:** 137.

Chen JC, Bongard F, Klein SR. A contemporary perspective on superior vena cava syndrome. *American Journal of Surgery*, 1990; **160:** 207.

Dartevelle P, Chapelier A, Navajas M. Replacement of the superior vena cava with polytetrafluoroethylene grafts combined with resection of mediastinal-pulmonary malignancy. *Journal of Thoracic and Cardiovascular Surgery*, 1987; **94:** 361.

Irving JD, Dondelinger RF, Reidy JF. Gianturco self-expanding stents: clinical experience in the vena cava and large veins. *Cardiovascular Interventional Radiology*, 1992; **15:** 319.

Related topics of interest

THORACIC INCISIONS

Sean Grondin, Michael R. Johnston

Throughout history surgeons have taught key technical points required to perform specific operative procedures. Perhaps the first and most crucial lesson for new surgeons is the importance of proper anatomic exposure to the success of a procedure and the ease in which it is completed. In thoracic surgery a thorough knowledge of the chest-wall anatomy is essential to facilitate proper exposure. Important anatomic structures to become familiar with include the thoracic cage and its musculature.

Thoracic cage

The thoracic cage consists of three bony elements which include the sternum anteriorly, the thoracic vertebrae posteriorly and 12 pairs of thoracic ribs connecting the two. The sternum is comprised of three structures; the bony manubrium superiorly, the body of the sternum and the cartilagenous xiphoid process inferiorly. The superior margin of the thoracic cage, termed the thoracic inlet, is bound by the manubrium anteriorly, the first thoracic rib laterally and the first thoracic vertebra posteriorly. Vital structures traversing this small, rigid opening include the trachea, esophagus, carotid arteries, jugular venous system and three major nerves; the phrenic, vagus and sympathetic trunk. The inferior margin on the thoracic cage is broad and compliant. It is bordered by the xiphoid process, the lower thoracic ribs with their costal cartilagenous margin and the 12th thoracic vertebra. The thorax is separated from the abdomen by the diaphragmatic muscle and tendon.

Thoracic cage musculature

The thoracic cage is supported by two layers of muscle. The intrinsic musculature consists primarily of the three intercostal muscle layers which are used for respiration and protection. The extrinsic musculature consists primarily of the pectoralis muscles, the serratus anterior muscle, the latissimus dorsi muscle as well as the sternocleidomastoid and the scalene muscles. The extrinsic group contributes to neck and pectoral girdle stabilization and mobilization of the upper limbs. Occasionally, the extrinsic musculature is used as accessory muscles of respiration.

Thoracic incisions

The choice of thoracic incision depends on the operation to be performed as well as the underlying pathology. Correlation with preoperative radiographic imaging is essential in planning surgery. The most common incisions utilized in thoracic surgery include:

- Median sternotomy.
- Posterolateral thoracotomy.
- Anterolateral thoracotomy.

- Axillary thoracotomy.
- Thoracoabdominal incision.
- Clamshell incision (bilateral anterior thoracotomies).
- VATS (video-assisted thoracoscopic surgery) incision.

Median sternotomy

1. *Indications.* Median sternotomy is currently the preferred incision for most cardiovascular procedures. Thoracic surgeons also use this incision for a variety of indications, including:

- Mediastinal tumor resection (e.g. thymoma).
- Bilateral lung volume reduction surgery/bullectomy.
- Resection of multiple pulmonary lesions (e.g. metastatectomy).
- Transpericardial access to trachea/bronchus (e.g. carinal tumors).
- Trauma.

2. *Operative technique.* The patient is placed in the supine position with a roll placed under the shoulders. A vertical incision is made from the sternal notch to the xyphoid process or upper abdomen, and the retrosternal space beneath the manubrium and the xyphoid process is mobilized. The pectoralis fascia is incised in the midline over the full length of the sternum and a mechanical saw is used to split the sternum in the midline. A sternal retractor is then placed and the incision opened slowly as the mediastinal connective tissue is divided. Following completion of the operation the sternum is reapproximated using stout stainless-steel wire and the pectoralis fascia is closed with a heavy absorbable suture.

3. *Advantage*
- Decreased postoperative pain since the incision is stable and no muscles are divided, leading to improved respiratory function and mobilization.

4. *Disadvantages*
- Sternal dehiscence (rare).
- Osteomyelitis occasionally requiring debridement with muscle advancement flap to repair .
- Posterior thoracic cavity, especially on left, is often difficult to access.

Posterolateral thoracotomy

1. *Indications.* This remains the most versatile incision used by the general thoracic surgeon. Indications include:

- Unilateral lung resection.
- Esophageal surgery.
- Chest-wall tumor resection.
- Unilateral lung volume reduction surgery/bullectomy.
- Tumors of the posterior mediastinum.

2. *Operative technique.* The patient is placed in the lateral decubitus position with careful attention to padding pressure points such as the elbows and knees, and the lateral position is maintained by adhesive tape, sand bags or a vacuum bean bag. The incision is made two fingerwidths below the tip of the scapula along the line of the ribs and can be extended posteriorly in a vertical direction between the scapula and the spine. The latissimus dorsi muscle is incised, whereas the serratus anterior muscle is preserved and retracted anteriorly. The ribs are counted in the subscapular space allowing the surgeon to identify the intercostal space of choice. Typically the fifth space is selected for lung resections, whereas the sixth or seventh interspace is chosen for esophageal surgery. The intercostal muscle and parietal pleura are divided along the inferior margin of the interspace to be entered. Some surgeons prefer to resect a portion of a rib to facilitate access to the thoracic cavity, especially in the elderly where brittle ribs are easily fractured by the chest retractor. A muscle-sparing variation of the posterolateral thoracotomy can be used for limited resections by raising skin flaps and extensive mobilization of the serratus anterior and latissimus dorsi muscles.

3. *Advantages*
- Good access to all regions of the thoracic cavity.
- Uncommon postoperative infections or herniation.

4. *Disadvantage*
- Increased postoperative pain secondary to muscle transection and/or displacement of the ribs.

Anterolateral thoracotomy

1. *Indications.* Anterolateral thoracotomy is used with decreasing frequency since better exposure is generally obtained with sternotomy or posterolateral thoracotomy. However, some surgeons prefer the anterolateral approach for specific indications such as:

- Open lung biopsy.
- Mobilization of the thoracic esophagus for resection.
- Lung resection.

2. *Operative technique.* The patient is placed in the supine position with a roll placed vertically under the back and pelvis to raise the operated side by about 45°. The ipsilateral arm is placed at the side. The incision is typically in the fourth or fifth intercostal space in the inframammary fold. The pectoralis muscles are divided and the intercostal muscles incised. A portion of costal cartilage may be removed to help gain extra exposure.

3. Advantages
- May save operative time by eliminating the need to reposition the patient during esophagogastrecomy.
- Fewer muscles to divide.

4. Disadvantages
- Limited exposure.
- Painful.
- Higher incidence of lung herniation since the intercostal space is more difficult to close.

Axillary thoracotomy

1. Indications. Although axillary thoracotomy is loosing favor to video-assisted thoracoscopic surgery, the following procedures can be performed via the axillary approach.

- Dorsal sympathectomy.
- First rib resection.
- Lung resection.
- Apical bullectomy.

2. Operative technique. The patient is placed in the lateral decubitus position, with the upper arm abducted 90° and the elbow flexed. The arm may be suspended or supported with an arm stand. An incision is made in the second intercostal space extending from the pectoralis major muscle anteriorly to the latissimus dorsi muscle posteriorly, below the hairline. The fibers of the serratus anterior muscle are split and the intercostal muscles divided.

3. Advantages
- Easy access since no major muscles are divided.
- Good exposure to upper thorax.
- Decreased postoperative discomfort.
- Incision hidden by the arm therefore cosmetically favorable.

4. Disadvantage
- Limited exposure to the lower thorax and mediastinum.
- Posterior extension of the incision may damage the long thoracic nerve.

Thoracoabdominal incision

1. Indications. The thoracoabdominal incision allows the surgeon to visualize both the pleural and peritoneal cavities with access to the organs and structures of the upper abdomen, lower chest and retroperitoneum. Thoracic surgeons use this incision for the following indications:

- Esophageal and gastric surgery.
- Retroperitoneal and diaphragmatic tumors.
- Surgery of the thoracic and upper abdominal aorta.

2. Operative technique. The patient is placed in the supine position with a roll beneath the left hip and shoulder. An incision is made overlying the interspace of choice (typically the sixth or seventh) and carried across the left upper quadrant of the abdomen obliquely. The costal margin is divided and the diaphragm circumferentially incised approximately 1 inch from its lateral margin to prevent phrenic nerve injury.

3. Advantage
- Excellent exposure.

4. Disadvantages
- Postoperative pain.
- Costochondritis can be a source of chronic pain in some patients.
- Diaphragmatic disfunction.

Clamshell incision (bilateral anterior thoracotomies)

1. Indications. Bilateral anterior thoracotomies provide maximum exposure to both hemithoraces and the mediastinal structures. Current indications include:

- Lung transplant surgery.
- Trauma.
- Bilateral lung resections.
- Lung volume reduction surgery.

2. Operative technique. The patient is placed in the supine position with a roll placed vertically along the upper thoracic spine. Bilateral anterior thoracotomy incisions are made in the inframammary fold along the fourth or fifth intercostal interspace. The pectoralis muscles are divided and the intercostal muscle incised. The internal mammary vein and artery are then ligated. A transverse sternal incision overlying the fourth intercostal space joins the two thoracotomy incisions. The thorax is opened using rib spreaders to allow the upper portion of the chest to be displaced caudally much like a 'clamshell' is opened. When closing the incision, care should be taken to realign and secure the sternum with wire sutures.

3. Advantage
- Excellent exposure.

4. Disadvantages
- Increased operative time.
- Occasional sternal instability.
- Persistent postoperative pain.

Further reading

Bains MS, Ginsberg RJ, Jones WG. The clamshell incision: an improved approach to bilateral pulmonary and mediastinal tumor. *Annals of Thoracic Surgery,* 1994; **58**: 30.

Ginsberg RJ. Alternative (muscle-sparing) incisions in thoracic surgery. *Annals of Thoracic Surgery,* 1993; **56:** 752.

Related topics of interest

THORACIC OUTLET SYNDROME

Chris Compeau, Michael R. Johnston

Thoracic outlet syndrome (syn. scalenus anticus, costoclavicular, hyperabduction, cervical rib or first thoracic rib syndromes) refers to symptoms arising from the compression of one or more of the major anatomic structures (i.e. the subclavian vessels, brachial plexus, sympathetic nerves) passing through the thoracic outlet. Compression usually occurs against the first rib or a cervical rib, if present.

Clincial presentation

The clinical presentation is extremely variable, depending on which structure (i.e. nerve or blood vessel) is compressed.

1. Nerve compression. The most frequent presenting symptom, it may be precipitated by exercise, trauma or rapid weight gain. Objective findings are usually minimal.

- Pain, paresthesias (95%), usually involving the ulnar nerve distribution in arm.
- Motor weakness, with atrophy of hypothenar and interosseus muscles (10%); rarely, clawing of the ring and little fingers.

2. Arterial compression
- Coldness, weakness and fatiguability of the arm and hand.
- Raynaud's phenomenon (<10%).
- Arterial occlusion may result in cold, cyanotic, ulcerated digits.

3. Venous compression
- Venous occlusion or obstruction is infrequent.
- 'Effort thrombosis' (Paget–Schroetter syndrome), comprises edema, venous distension and discoloration of the upper limb.

Investigations

Specific physical maneuvers (i.e. Adson, costoclavicular, hyperabduction and modified Roos tests) are designed to reproduce the symptoms, and to demonstrate loss or decrease of the radial pulse. Clinical sensory testing (pressure, vibration, two-point discrimination) and provocative tests (i.e. Tinel's sign) are used to document neurological defects. Objective studies to measure nerve conduction velocity (i.e. nerve conduction studies) are generally difficult to standardize, perform and reproduce. Values of less than 70 m/second suggest neurovascular compression across the thoracic outlet. Further reduction in conduction velocity may be used to grade severity. Radiographic studies (i.e. CXR, cervical spine, CT, MRI) may demonstrate cervical ribs, degenerative vertebral changes and intervertebral narrowing. Arteriography and venography may demonstrate atheromatous plaques, localized areas of stenosis or compression, and post-stenotic dilation.

Differential diagnosis

The difficulty in making a definitive diagnosis of thoracic outlet syndrome requires the surgeon to be familiar with a wide differential diagnosis.

1. *Neurologic disorders*
- Cervical spine: herniated disk, degenerative disease, arthritis, tumor.
- Brachial plexus: post-traumatic injury, Pancoast tumor.
- Peripheral nerves: entrapment syndromes, neuropathies, tumor, trauma.

2. *Vascular*
- Arterial: atheroma, thrombosis, aneurysm, embolus, reflex vasomotor dystrophy, vasculitis, collagen disorders.
- Venous: thrombophlebitis, SVCO.

3. *Miscellaneous*
- Angina, esophageal or pulmonary causes.

Management

1. *Nonoperative*
- Patient education, modify activities which precipitate symptoms.
- Physiotherapy, to improve posture, cervicothoracic muscle-strengthing exercises.
- Subclavian vein thrombosis: anticoagulation, thrombolysis, compression garment, arm elevation.
- Weight loss if the patient is obese.

2. *Surgery.* This is indicated in patients with thoracic outlet syndrome not relieved by conservative measures (about 5% of patients). The decision to operate (or not) may also be influenced by the psychiatric overlay that often accompanies the syndrome and medico-legal considerations.

Transaxillary first rib resection to 'decompress' the thoracic outlet, including division of any associated fibrous bands and excision of a compressive cervical rib, is the preferred approach initially. This results in a 90% improvement of symptoms. Recurrence occurs with failure to remove sufficient first rib or with postoperative scarring. Concurrent dorsal sympathectomy is rarely necessary. The supraclavicular approach may also be used, especially if extensive neurolysis, or division of anterior fibrous bands, is warranted. The posterior approach is reserved for reoperation. This approach provides excellent exposure of nerve roots and the brachial plexus, and permits wide exposure of the posterior first rib remnant. Dorsal sympathectomy to remove the T1–3 ganglia (preserving C8 to avoid Horner's syndrome), is recommended for associated causalgia-like symptoms, sympathetic-related pain or Raynaud's phenomenon.

Further reading

Cheng SWK, Stoney RJ. Supraclavicular reoperation for neurogenic thoracic outlet syndrome. *Journal of Vascular Surgery,* 1994; **19:** 565.

Mackinnon S, Patterson GA, Urschel HC. Thoracic outlet syndromes. In: Pearson FG, Deslauriers J, Ginsberg RJ, Hiebert CA, McKneally MF, Urschel HC, eds. *Thoracic Surgery.* New York: Churchill Livingstone, 1995; 1211.

Roos DB. Transaxillary approach for first rib resection to relieve thoracic outlet syndrome. *Annals of Surgery,* 1966; **163:** 354.

Urschel HC. Dorsal sympathectomy and management of thoracic outlet syndrome with VATS. *Annals of Thoracic Surgery,* 1993; **56:** 717.

Urschel HC, Razzuk MA, Wood RE, Paulson DL. Objective diagnosis (ulnar nerve conduction velocity) and current therapy of the thoracic outlet syndrome. *Annals of Thoracic Surgery,* 1971; **12:** 608.

Related topic of interest

THYMOMA

Gail Darling

Thymoma is the most common tumor of the anterior mediastinum, but is still exceedingly rare in clinical practice with an incidence of 0.10–0.18 per 100 000. Twelve percent of patients with myasthenia gravis have an associated thymoma and about 30–50% of patients with thymoma are found to have myasthenia gravis.

Signs and symptoms

Thirty percent of cases are asymptomatic and 30% have cough, dyspnea and chest pain. Muscle fatigue characteristic of myasthenia gravis (MG) occurs in 35–65%, and neck and facial swelling from superior venal cava syndrome in 3–5%. Symptoms of other autoimmune disorders occur in 1–11%, including:

- Bacterial infections and diarrhea from hypogammaglobulinemia.
- Fatigue and anemia from pure red cell aplasia.
- Blisters and superficial skin erosions indicative of pemphagus foliaceus.
- Rapidly progressive congestive heart failure from giant cell myocarditis.

Investigations

- Chest CT should be performed with intravenous contrast in all patients with a suspected mediastinal mass or MG.
- MRI offers no advantage.
- Serum levels of βHCG and α-fetoprotein to aid in the diagnosis of a germ cell tumor.
- Acetycholine receptor antibody levels, single fiber EMG and Tensilon test for suspected MG.
- Radioisotope thyroid scan if substernal goiter is suspected.

Diagnosis

Thymoma may be strongly suspected by the radiographic appearance of a solitary anterior mediastinal mass without evidence of adenopathy or thyroid involvement.

Biopsy (needle or core vs. open). The role of needle biopsy for a suspected thymoma is controversial. Disadvantages include failure to yield a definitive diagnosis or to differentiate benign from malignant thymoma and the risk of seeding tumor cells in the mediastinum or pleural space ('drop metastases'). Currently, pathologists can usually differentiate thymoma from lymphoma, germ cell or other tumors but still can not tell if the thymoma is benign or malignant.

- Open biopsy via anterior mediastinotomy (Chamberlain procedure) usually gives sufficient tissue, but seeding into the operative site and violation of the tumor capsule are major concerns.

- Diagnostic accuracy is 59% for needle biopsy and 81% for open biopsy. Preoperative biopsy is recommended if the tumor appears to invade mediastinal structures, appears unresectable, if there are pleural or pericardial effusions or the clinical presentation is suggestive of lymphoma or other non-thymomatous tumors.

Classification

(a) Based on predominant cell type:

- Epithelial predominant (most aggressive).
- Lymphocytic.
- Mixed.
- Spindle cell.

(b) Based on the histological similarity to normal thymus (Muller Hermalink classification):

- Cortical.
- Medullary.
- Mixed.

Staging

Modified Masoaka staging system:

- Stage I: no invasion of capsule microscopically or macroscopically.
- Stage II: microscopic or macroscopic invasion of the capsule or invasion into mediastinal fat or pleura.
- Stage III: invasion of mediastinal structures: lung, great vessels, pericardium.
- Stage IVa: pleural or pericardial metastases (drop metastases).
- Stage IVb: distant metastases.

Stage at presentation:

- 53% stage I.
- 27% stage II.
- 16% stage III.
- 4% stage IV.

Management

- Stage I: total thymectomy.
- Stage II: total thymectomy plus postoperative radiation (RT).
- Stage III: total thymectomy and resection of all nonvital structures invaded by the tumor (i.e. pericardium, lung, innominate vein, etc.) plus postoperative radiation (chemotherapy is optional). If the tumor appears unresectable, chemotherapy and radiation should be followed by surgical debulking.
- Stage IVa: chemotherapy followed by resection of the primary tumor and drop metastases with postoperative radiation to mediastinum.
- Stage IVb: chemotherapy.

Role of surgery

- Primary treatment of stage I and II tumors.
- Usual approach is through either partial or complete sternotomy.
- VATS approach is experimental and can not be currently recommended.
- Complete thymectomy with margins of normal tissue around tumor.
- Avoid injury to phrenic nerves, but if the only obstacle to a complete resection is invasion into one phrenic nerve, it can be sacrificed as long as the other nerve is preserved.
- Role of tumor debulking:
  - (a) Controversial but appears to be beneficial.
  - (b) Five-year survival is 28–78% for debulking vs. 0–40% with biopsy only. The difference may be related to case selection, rather than surgery.

Role of radiation

- Thymoma is very radiosensitive.
- Recurrence rate is 5% in completely resected stage II and stage III tumors if postoperative radiation is given, vs. 28% recurrence without radiation. No difference in survival has been noted.
- A suitable dose is 40–55 Gy.

Role of chemotherapy

- Very chemosensitive.
- The best regimen and exact role are still to be defined.
- Response rates up to 84% with cisplatin-based regimens.
- Complete remissions: 10–68%.

Recurrence

- Stage is the only independent predictor: stage I: <5%; stage II: 5–20%; stage III: 15–30%; stage IV: 25–55%.
- Mean time to recurrence is 5.5 years, with a range of 0–16 years.
- Intrathoracic recurrence is 70–80%.
- Treatment: reresection, chemotherapy, RT.

Prognosis

- Independent predictors of survival include completeness of surgical resection; stage; histology (epithelial predominant is worst, lymphocytic and spindle cell are best); size >11 cm predicts poor prognosis).
- MG is not a prognostic factor.
- Survival rates for each stage are given in *Table 1*.

Cause of death

- Unrelated to tumor: 65%.
- Progressive disease: 35%.
- Associated autoimmune disease: 25%.

Table 1. Survival from thymoma

Stage	Survival (%)		
	5 year	10 year	15 year
I	85	80	75
II	75	60	70
III	70	55	30
IV	50	30	8

Further reading

Blumberg D, Port JL, Weksler B, Delgado R, Rosai J, Bains MS, Ginsberg RJ, Martini N, McCormack PM, Rusch V, Burt ME. Thymoma: a multivariate analysis of factors predicting survival. *Annals of Thoracic Surgery*, 1995; **60:** 908.

Ferguson MK. Transcervical thymectomy. *Chest Surgery Clinics of North America*, 1996; **6:** 105.

Kohman LJ. Controversies in the management of malignant thymoma. *Chest*, 1997; **112 (Suppl.):** 296S.

McCart JA, Gaspar L, Inculet R, Casson AG. Predictors of survival following surgical resection of thymoma. *Journal of Surgical Oncology*, 1993; **54:** 233.

Wilkins EW, Grillo HC, Scannell G, Moncure AC, Mathieson DJ. Role of staging in prognosis and management of thymoma. *Annals of Thoracic Surgery*, 1991; **51:** 888.

Related topics of interest

Mediastinum and mediastinal masses (p. 170)
Superior vena cava syndrome (p. 232)

TRACHEAL RESECTION

Shaf Keshafjee, Hani K. Najm

Prior to the 1960s tracheal resection and reconstruction by primary anastomosis was limited to anecdotal reports, as it was generally assumed that no more than 3–4 tracheal rings (i.e. up to 3 cm) could be resected and reanastomosed. With the advent of endotracheal intubation and mechanical ventilation, there was a surge in the incidence of postintubation injuries. This stimulated the development of new techniques for safe tracheal resection and reconstruction utilizing neck flexion and various release maneuvers. In most patients approximately half of the trachea can be safely resected with a primary reconstruction. Experience and a thorough knowledge of tracheal anatomy, blood supply and surgical techniques are mandatory before contemplating this type of surgery, especially for resections of the upper or lower ends of the trachea, which may pose a specific technical challenge.

Indications
- Postintubation stricture.
- Symptomatic tracheal stenosis (i.e. idiopathic, extrinsic compression).
- Benign or malignant tracheal tumors.
- Some congenital anomalies (i.e. vascular rings).

Anatomy of the adult trachea
- Generally 11 cm long (10–13 cm); 18–22 rings (about 2 rings per cm).
- 2.3 cm wide by 1.8 cm anteroposterior diameter.
- The trachea shortens with age.

1. Anatomic relationships
- Superior: vocal cords (1.5–2 cm above the first ring).
- Anterior: thyroid isthmus (second or third ring), innominate artery, aortic arch.
- Posterior: esophagus, separated by an avascular plane of connective tissue.
- Lateral: azygous veins, pleura, recurrent laryngeal nerves.
- Inferior: anterior and posterior subcarnial lymph nodes.

2. Arterial blood supply. The arterial blood supply is segmental, from adjacent vessels which also supply the mediastinal viscera including the esophagus. The trachea is generally supplied by up to three branches from the inferior thyroid artery, and to a variable extent from the subclavian, superior intercostal, internal thoracic and middle bronchial arteries. An extensive network of lateral longitudinal collaterals exists, which penetrate between the cartilagenous rings to supply the submucosa.

Essential information required before surgical resection
- Anatomic location: proximal and distal extent of lesion (rigid bronchoscopy).
- Amount of uninvolved airway (rigid bronchoscopy).
- Extension to surrounding structures (CT scanning).

- Evidence of metastasis (staging, CT scanning).
- Glottic function (direct or indirect laryngoscopy).

Surgical technique

1. *Anesthetic considerations*
- Sterile anesthetic ventilator circuits.
- Uncut cuffed armored endotracheal tube of sufficient length to intubate main stem bronchi.
- Jet ventilation vs. intermittent intubation.
- Planned awake extubation in the operating room.

2. *Approach*
- Upper-third: cervical collar incision with or without complete or partial sternal split.
- Mid-third:
  Cervical and full sternotomy
  Possible transpericardial approach
  'Trap door' incision through the right fourth intercostal space.
- Lower-third: right thoracotomy.
- Carina:
  Right thoracotomy
  Median sternotomy
  Bilateral transverse thoracotomy ('clamshell' incision).

3. *Strategy*
- Preserve blood supply to trachea through the lateral vascular pedicles.
- Allow 1 cm margin from gross tumor if possible.
- Check frozen section of resection margins. Occasionally it may be necessary to accept microscopic positive margins, rather than to extend the resection judged to be safe.
- Choice of release maneuver is done after resection.
- Generally up to 4–5 cm can be resected with no release maneuver.

4. *Release maneuvers (to decrease tension on the tracheal anastomosis)*
- Pretracheal dissection.
- Cervical flexion (guardian chin stitch).
- Laryngeal release procedures (not used in carinal resection).
  Suprahyoid (Montgomery). Divide mylohyoid, geniohyoid and genioglossus muscles and the two horns of hyoid bone to give 2 cm extra length.
  Infrahyoid (Dedo). Divide thyrohyoid muscle on both sides, thyrohyoid membrane and ligament, preserving the submucosal plexus and avoiding damage to the superior laryngeal nerve. Gives 1–2 cm extra length. Aspiration can be a significant problem after surgery.

- Hilar release: A 'U'-shaped incision in the pericardium beneath the inferior pulmonary vein or complete circular incision of the pericardium around the hilum.

5. *Anastomotic technique*
- Apply heavy traction sutures laterally above and below the anastomotic site.
- Interrupted 3/0 or 4/0 absorable sutures (knots tied on outside) or fine stainless-steel wires (knots should be inside).
- Avoid tension.
- Intrathoracic anastomoses are covered with pedicled pleura, pericardial fat or mobilized gastrocolic omentum. Cervical anastomosis may be covered with a pedicled strap muscle flap or mobilized thyroid isthmus.

6. *Adjunctive maneuvers.* Recurrent laryngeal nerves should be preserved carefully unless involved with tumor. The left nerve runs in the tracheoesophageal groove for almost the entire length of the trachea, whereas the right nerve approaches the trachea laterally. Both nerves pass deep into the cricothyroid muscle and posterior to the cricothyroid articulations. Above this level the nerves enter the larynx medial to the inferior cornua of the thyroid cartilage. Involved lymph nodes should be removed *en bloc* taking care not to devascularize the remaining trachea. Tumors involving the subglottic airway may be managed by circumferential resection of the distal cricoid, preserving the posterior perichondrium or a thin shell of the posterior cricoid plate, to maintain laryngeal and vocal function.

Complications

1. *Early*
- Airway obstruction, anastomotic edema. May require re-intubation with a deflated or uncuffed endotracheal tube. Tracheostomy is now rarely necessary. The airway is reassessed bronchoscopically (local anesthesia) in the operating room after 2–3 days.
- Recurrent laryngeal nerve injury (transient or permanent).
- Air leak, subcutaneous emphysema.
- Aspiration, dyscoordinated swallowing. Semi-solids are started on the second postoperative day, and are generally better tolerated than liquids.
- Anastomotic dehiscence.
- Bleeding.
- Infection, abscess.

2. *Late*
- Restenosis.
- Suture-line granuloma.
- Tracheoesophageal fistula.
- Tracheoinnominate artery fistula.

Further reading

Dedo HH, Fishman NH. Laryngeal release and sleeve resection for tracheal stenosis. *Annals of Otology, Rhinology and Laryngology,* 1969; **78:** 285.

Grillo HC, Mathisen DJ, Wain JC. Laryngotracheal resection and reconstruction for subglottic stenosis. *Annals of Thoracic Surgery,* 1992; **53:** 54.

Keshafjee S, Pearson FG. Tracheal resection. In: Pearson FG, Deslauriers J, Ginsberg RJ, Hiebert CA, McKneally MF, Urschel HC, eds. *Thoracic Surgery.* New York: Churchill Livingstone, 1995; 333.

Montgomery WW. The surgical management of supraglottic and subglottic stenosis. *Annals of Otology, Rhinology and Laryngology,* 1968; **77:** 534.

Related topics of interest

TRACHEAL STENOSIS

Shaf Keshafjee, Hani K. Najm

Tracheal stenosis usually implies a discrete narrowing of part of the trachea, most commonly a result of postintubation injury.

Classification and etiology: congenital

1. Webs and diaphragms

2. Stenosis. Results from a developmental defect in which the membranous trachea is deficient, and the wall consists of complete (or almost complete) cartilagenous rings. Often associated with other anomalies of the tracheobronchial tree, including a pulmonary artery sling, aberrant right middle and lower lobe bronchi arising from the left mainstem bronchus and unilateral pulmonary agenesis. Three patterns are described:

- Generalized hypoplasia.
- Funnel-like narrowing.
- Segmental stenosis.

3. Tracheomalacia. Decreased rigidity of the trachea due to a structural abnormality of its wall. This results in a generalized narrowing and collapse of the airway during ventilation (expiration) or swallowing. Associated with esophageal atresia, and rarely compression from vascular rings, other mediastinal structures or postoperatively.

Classification and etiology: acquired

1. Postintubation. Initial mucosal injury may occur as early as 4 hours after intubation, resulting in mucosal ulceration, with exposure of tracheal cartilage. Following extubation, these devitalized areas heal by fibrosis and stricture. Full-thickness injury may result in a tracheoesophageal or tracheoinominate artery fistula.

2. Post-traumatic. Resulting from avulsion of the trachea from the larynx; partial or complete fracture of the mediastinal trachea.

3. Postinfectious. Usually associated with tuberculosis or diphtheria.

4. Neoplastic. Benign and malignant tumors.

5. Miscellaneous
- Fibrosing mediastinitis.
- Wegener's granulomatosis.
- Amyloidosis.

- Idiopathic. A circumferential fibrotic stenosis of the sub-glottic larynx or upper trachea, with a normal distal trachea. Usually 2 cm in length, narrowing the lumen to 2 mm. Histologically the fibrosis is keloidal (eosinophilic collagen), and replaces the lamina propia. The tracheal mucosa usually shows squamous metaplasia. The etiology of this lesion is unknown, and its natural history is of progression.

Clinical presentation

1. History and examination. Patients often present with gradually worsening airway obstruction (dyspnea, wheeze, 'asthma') and a previous history of trauma or intubation. Acute airway obstruction occurs when the tracheal lumen reaches a critical diameter, or becomes obstructed by a mucus plug or foreign body. Physical examination may reveal stridor and a healed tracheostomy site.

2. Radiology. Standard posterior–anterior and lateral films of chest, or lateral neck X-rays, may occasionally reveal abnormalities of the airway. These are better evaluated by linear tomography (if available). CT scanning, especially spiral CT with reconstruction, has become the investigation of choice. MRI remains an underused investigation. Bronchography is now rarely used.

3. Bronchoscopy. Rigid and flexible techniques are complementary, and are essential to obtain the diagnosis (i.e. malignant vs. benign) and for planning surgery (i.e. location of stenosis, length of stricture, relation to vocal cords and carina, associated destruction of cartilage, presence of infection). Critical airway stenosis should be managed by the use of the rigid bronchoscope for airway control, and dilation of the stricture (especially if <6 mm) while planning definitive therapy.

4. Pulmonary function studies. Flow volume loops may help determine the extent of respiratory impairment (flattening of inspiratory and expiratory curves), and may be used to document improvement after surgery.

Intubation injury

1. Endotracheal tube injuries
- Vocal cords: granuloma, stenosis.
- Cuff sites: stenosis, tracheoesophageal fistula.
- Tube tip site: granuloma, esophageal or inominate arterial fistula.

2. Cuffed tracheostomy tube injuries
- Stomal site: anterior stenosis, granuloma, malacia.
- Cuff site: stenosis, tracheoesophageal fistula.
- Tube tip site: granuloma, esophageal or inominate artery fistula.

Management

1. General. Coexisting disorders should be treated, particularly pulmonary infections, protein depletion and malnutrition.

2. Dilatation. Rigid bronchoscope and gum tip bougies. Keep the patient breathing spontaneously until an airway is secured.

3. Dilatation with stenting. Used as a temporizing measure. Silastic T-tubes, T-Y tubes or expandable metal stents are used. The stent tip should be well below the stenotic area. This may be a definitive treatment for patients unable to undergo resection.

4. Resection and primary reconstruction. Definitive management for most patients, assuming satisfactory anesthetic risk. The majority of patients (>90%) will achieve good/satisfactory results in terms of breathing, voice and swallowing. Optimal results are obtained by experienced surgeons in centers with a particular interest in airway surgery, where mortality approximates 3%.

5. Tracheostomy. Now rarely used as permanent therapy.

6. Laser. Not a recommended treatment (temporary or permanent) for benign tracheal stenoses since the laser causes further injury to the airway. This may preclude successful surgical resection and reconstruction.

Further reading

Grillo HC, Donahue DM, Mathisen DJ. Postintubation tracheal stenosis: treatment and results. *Journal of Thoracic and Cardiovascular Surgery,* 1995; **109:** 486.
Grillo HC, Mack EJ, Mathisen DJ, Wain JC. Idiopathic laryngotracheal stenosis and its management. *Annals of Thoracic Surgery,* 1993; **56:** 80.
Lobe TE. Congenital tracheal stenosis. *Chest Surgery Clinics of North America,* 1993; **3:** 495.

Related topics of interest

TRACHEAL TUMORS

Shaf Keshafjee, Hani K. Najm

Primary tracheal tumors are rare; secondary tumors are more common. Most primary tumors in adults are malignant, whereas in children they tend to be benign. In general the incidence is equally distributed between males and females. Primary malignant tumors of the trachea represent about 2% of all upper-airway tumors.

Primary tumors

1. Benign. May arise from any component of the tracheal wall, and account for over 90% of primary tumors in children. Fewer than 10% of adult tumors are benign.

- Squamous papilloma. The most common benign tumor. Usually multifocal throughout the tracheobronchial tree, and may regress after puberty.
- Pleomorphic adenoma.
- Granular cell tumor.
- Leiomyoma.
- Chondroma.
- Paraganglioma.
- Vascular malformation (i.e. hemangioma).

2. Intermediate
- Carcinoid.
- Mucoepidermoid.
- Pseudosarcoma.

3. Malignant. Over 90% of adult tumors are malignant, the most common being squamous cell carcinoma and adenoid cystic tumors.

- Squamous cell carcinoma occurs commonly in males, with a similar age distribution to non-small cell lung cancer, and is associated with cigarette smoking. Tumors may be exophytic or ulcerative, and regional lymph-node metastases are common. Most tumors are locally advanced at presentation. Multiple primary tumors of the upper aerodigestive tract (i.e. oropharynx, lung, esophagus) are common.
- Adenoid cystic carcinoma was previously referred to as 'cylindroma'. It affects males and females of all ages. It is a slow-growing tumor, with extensive local invasion beyond the visible and palpable tumor, and the overlying tracheal mucosa often appears intact. Submucosal spread occurs longitudinally and circumferentially and mediastinal structures are displaced rather than invaded. Regional lymph node metastasis is seen in fewer than 10% of patients. Distant metastases are uncommon, although the lung is the commonest site. Other malignant tumors include:

Small cell carcinoma.
Atypical carcinoma.
Melanoma.
Spindle cell sarcoma.
Rhabdomyosarcoma.
Malignant fibrous histocytoma.

Secondary tumors

Local invasion from primary tumors of the:
- Larynx.
- Thyroid.
- Lung.
- Esophagus.

Metastasis to trachea (i.e. renal cell carcinoma, melanoma, thyroid carcinoma), or to the mediastinum with secondary invasion of trachea (i.e. carcinoma of the breast).

Clinical presentation

- Airway obstruction (i.e. dyspnea, wheezing and stridor).
- Mucosal irritation and ulceration (i.e. cough, hemoptysis).
- Direct invasion of contiguous structures (i.e. esophagus producing dysphagia, recurrent laryngeal nerve producing hoarseness).
- Distant metastases.

It should be noted that patients may be misdiagnosed with asthma or chronic bronchitis long before the correct diagnosis is made. Plain CXR usually show clear lung fields, with only subtle tracheal or mediastinal abnormalities.

Diagnosis and staging

1. Endoscopy. Flexible bronchoscopy through an endotracheal tube may miss proximal tracheal tumors. Rigid bronchoscopy is essential for a complete examination of the trachea, to maintain safe control of the airway and to allow accurate assessment of potential resectability. Adequate biopsies should be taken for histopathology. Esophagoscopy should also be performed in patients with dysphagia, or if the tumor is extensive.

2. Radiology
- Tracheal tomography.
- CT scan (with 3-D reconstruction of airway) provides excellent anatomical delineation of airway pathology.
- MRI is still under review as an imaging modality for airway tumors.
- Contrast studies of the esophagus are useful in selected patients; bronchography is rarely used.

3. Pulmonary function studies. Flow–volume loops may demonstrate flattening of inspiratory and expiratory curves suggesting a fixed upper-airway obstruction.

Management	As most malignant tracheal tumors are locally advanced at presentation, palliative approaches to preserve the airway are indicated. However, the definitive treatment of a well-localized tracheal tumor is surgical resection, provided there are no distant metastases (a relative contraindication for adenoidcystic carcinomas), no direct invasion of mediastinal structures and acceptable anesthetic risk.

1. Surgery
- Resection and primary reconstruction. See 'Tracheal resection', p. 248.
- Laryngotracheal resections with or without cervico-mediastinal exenteration.
- Staged reconstruction.
- Stenting: T-tube, T-Y tube or tracheostomy. See 'Stents: airway', p. 230.
- Endoscopic palliative resection ('coring-out', laser).

2. Radiotherapy. Indicated for the palliative therapy of unresectable tumors. However, mucosal edema may result in airway obstruction. This modality should therefore be combined with endoscopic debridement (or stenting) in patients with critical airway obstruction. Radiotherapy is widely recommended as adjuvant therapy after resection of adenoid cystic and squamous cell carcinomas. However, this has not been evaluated in a randomized clinical trial. There has been increased recent interest in brachytherapy and high-dose (curative) external-beam therapy for small lesions (especially at the carina).

3. Chemotherapy. A lack of active agents, and relatively limited patient numbers have generally precluded clinical trials to evaluate the role of of chemotherapy or combined modality therapy (i.e. chemoradiotherapy).

Outcome

One-third of patients will have unresectable tumor and should be treated with radiotherapy, tracheostomy or stent; one-third will be resectable but without possibility for reconstruction; and one-third will be resectable with primary reconstruction. Surgical mortality is 5–10%. This ranges from 1–3% for tracheal resection to 10–20% for carinal resection. It should be noted that only a few centers in the world have reported a significant experience with surgical resection of primary tracheal tumors. Ten-year survival for squamous cell carcinoma is 33%, 10-year survival for adenoidcystic carcinoma is 45% (even with positive resection margins).

Further reading

Grillo HC, Mathisen DJ. Primary tracheal tumors: treatment and results. *Annals of Thoracic Surgery,* 1990; **49:** 69.

Pearson FG, Cardoso P, Keshafjee S. Upper airway tumors. In: Pearson FG, Deslauriers J, Ginsberg RJ, Hiebert CA, McKneally MF, Urschel HC, eds. *Thoracic Surgery.* New York: Churchill Livingstone, 1995; 285.

Shankar S, George PJ, Hetzel MR, Goldstraw P. Elective resection of tumors of the trachea and main carina after endoscopic laser therapy. *Thorax,* 1990; **45:** 493.

Related topics of interest

TRACHEOESOPHAGEAL AND TRACHEOINOMINATE ARTERY FISTULAE

Shaf Keshafjee, Hani K. Najm

Destruction of the posterior membraneous trachea may result in the development of a fistula from the airway to the esophagus. Previously it was often due to granulomatous diseases, but in recent years, the most common cause is neoplastic, or as a result of prolonged intubation. Full-thickness erosion of the anterior tracheal wall may result in the uncommon, but often lethal, tracheoinominate artery fistula.

Tracheoesophageal fistula

Classification and etiology

1. *Congenital.* Tracheoesophageal fistula with or without esophageal atresia.

2. *Acquired*
- Inflammatory (i.e. tuberculosis, histoplasmosis).
- Traumatic (i.e. blunt or penetrating injury).
- Postintubation. Airway and esophagus: the combination of a cuffed endotracheal tube and nasogastric tube is the most common cause.
- Neoplastic. Tumors of the airway or esophagus (most common).

Clinical presentation

Evidence of gastric content in the airway or a marked increase in tracheal secretions is suggestive. In ventilated patients, if the cuff of the endotracheal tube (or tracheostomy) is above the fistula, gastric distention will occur. The diagnosis is confirmed easily by direct visualization at bronchoscopy or esophagoscopy. In patients with esophageal tumors, the diagnosis may be made (inadvertently) at the time of barium swallow, when the fistula and a bronchogram will be readily seen. In this situation, aspiration of barium is preferable to hyperosmolar, water-soluble contrast agents which may result in pneumonitis.

Management

1. *Benign tracheoesophageal fistula.* Conservative management until the patient is weaned off the ventilator is preferred to attempts at repair in a ventilated patient. The nasogastric tube is removed and a gastrostomy placed to decompress the stomach and minimize gastroesophageal reflux. A jejunostomy tube is placed for feeding. The primary treatment is repair and/or resection of the tracheal disruption and closure of the esophageal defect. It is rare that the fistula can be closed primarily. A vascularized pedicle (i.e. muscle flap, omentum) is

interposed between the suture lines. If esophageal resection is required, upper GI continuity is restored by reconstruction using stomach or colon.

2. Malignant tracheoesophageal fistula. Generally associated with poor prognosis (survival measured in weeks). Therefore, palliative esophageal intubation (stent) to decrease soiling of airway is indicated. In selected patients, esophageal diversion with an extra-anatomic bypass (such as a substernal gastric bypass) to prevent airway soiling may be considered.

Tracheoinominate artery fistula

Etiology

Most commonly results from full-thickness erosion of the anterior tracheal wall with fistularization to the inominate artery.

1. Intubation injury
- Low placement of a tracheostomy (i.e. stoma below the second or third tracheal ring).
- Hyperinflation of a tracheostomy or endotracheal tube cuff.
- An abnormally high inominate artery.
- Prolonged intubation, even with a normally placed tracheostomy.

2. Postoperative. Reported following tracheal resection, or extended laryngectomy, especially in a previously irradiated field, in the presence of infection and when vascularized tissue has not been interposed between the artery and the airway.

Diagnosis

Massive bleeding. Premonitory bleeding around the tracheostomy site, through the tracheostomy tube, or through the mouth or nose, may preceed massive bleeding, and therefore a high index of suspicion should be maintained.

Management

1. Herald bleed. Often a brisk, but self-limiting bleeding episode occurs within the airway. In a patient at risk this should immediately raise the possiblility of a tracheoinominate fistula. Flexible bronchoscopy is indicated to define the source of bleeding. The cuff of the tracheostomy tube or endotracheal tube should be deflated and withdrawn carefully to visualize the airway fully. The bronchoscope should also be introduced transnasally to examine the oropharynx and airway above the cuff. If a fistula is suspected, the neck is explored in the operating room. An upper sternotomy may be required for access and vascular control. In the presence of a fistula, inominate artery resection is advised. Vascular bypass is not necessary. As the operative site is generally contaminated, interposition of healthy, vascularized tissue (i.e. muscle flap, omentum) is advised. Attempts to repair the artery generally fail, even with the interposition of healthy tissues. The tracheal defect may be closed directly if small and sufficient healthy tissues are available to cover the repair. Otherwise, the defect is packed open (secondary closure). The airway is maintained by endotracheal intubation with the balloon positioned above the tracheal repair or defect. Occasionally jet ventilation may be required.

2. *Massive bleed.* This is the usual presentation, and immediate management requires simultaneous control of the airway and control of bleeding. The following maneuvers may be useful:

- Hyperinflate the tracheostomy balloon and direct the tip anteriorly to compress the artery.
- Pass an endotracheal tube, remove the tracheostomy and advance the endotracheal tube across the fistula into the distal airway. The inominate artery is compressed against the manubrium by a finger inserted through the tracheostome.
- A rigid bronchoscope may be used to compress the inominate artery against the sternum, while providing access to the airway.

With the airway secure and bleeding controlled, the patient is taken to the operating room for further resuscitation and definitive management (as outlined above).

Further reading

Deslauriers J, Ginsberg RJ, Nelems JM, Pearson FG. Inomonate artery rupture: a major complication of tracheal surgery. *Annals of Thoracic Surgery,* 1975; **20:** 671.

Kotsis L, Zubovits K, Vadasz P. Management of malignant tracheoesophageal fistulas with a cuffed funnel tube. *Annals of Thoracic Surgery,* 1997; **64:** 355.

Low DE, Kozarek RA. Comparison of conventional and wire mesh expandable prostheses and surgical bypass in patients with malignant esophagorespiratory fistulae. *Annals of Thoracic Surgery,* 1998; **65:** 919.

Mathisen DJ, Grillo HC, Wain JC. Management of acquired nonmalignant tracheoesophageal fistula. *Annals of Thoracic Surgery,* 1991; **52:** 759.

Related topics of interest

TRACHEOSTOMY

Alan G. Casson

Despite several recent modifications (i.e. percutaneous tracheostomy, minitracheostomy) or variations (i.e. cricothyroidotomy), a surgical tracheostomy continues to provide reliable access to the airway.

Indications

- Upper airway obstruction.
- Tracheobronchial toilet.
- Airway access for mechanical ventilation.
- Elimination of dead space.

Technique

An elective tracheostomy is performed under optimal conditions in the operating room, with adequate lighting, instruments, suction, etc. Alternative settings include the intensive care unit or at the bedside. The technique may be performed under local or general anesthesia. The patient is positioned with the neck hyperextended, and a transverse skin incision one fingerwidth below the cricoid is used, and dissection continued in the midline (avascular). The thyroid isthmus is retracted superiorly or inferiorly, and rarely requires division. A cricoid hook is used to stabilize the trachea. Alternatively, a heavy traction suture can be placed around the first tracheal ring and tied outside the wound. This is left in place until the stoma has matured as an aid to reinserting a dislodged tube. A vertical incision of the second and third tracheal rings is used (minimal residual tracheal damage), although several variations exist, each with personal preference. A tracheostomy tube of appropiate size is inserted with the obturator in place and the cuff deflated. Once the tracheostomy tube is in place, the obturator is removed and a suction catheter introduced through the tube. Free passage into the lower airway and the aspiration of tracheal secretions confirms proper placement. If the catheter does not pass easily beyond the tip of the tube, the tube may be lying in the pretracheal space and should be removed and reinserted. After ensuring proper placement, the cuff is inflated and the inner cannula placed prior to ventilation. The tube is sutured to the skin and a tracheostomy tape tied around the neck to prevent dislodgement in the early postoperative period.

Complications

1. Intraoperative
- Bleeding.
- Pneumothorax.
- Hypoxia leading to cardiorespiratory arrest. Usually this is a result of unrecognized misplacement of the tracheostomy tube into the pretracheal space.

2. *Postoperative*
- Bleeding.
- Wound infection.
- Tube obstruction or displacement.
- Swallowing difficulty.
- Tracheal stenosis.
- Tracheoesophageal fistula.
- Tracheoinominate artery fistula.
- Tracheocutaneous fistula.

Percutaneous tracheostomy

Widespread use of this technique by a range of physicians resulted in reports of significant complications, including false passage, pneumothorax, bleeding, esophageal injury and death. Under controlled, elective conditions, it is a quick, efficient and relatively inexpensive technique to obtain a surgical airway, especially when performed by an operator familiar with conventional tracheostomy. Several kits are now available commercially, comprising a guidewire and a range of dilators. This technique should not be used to establish an emergency airway.

Minitracheostomy

This technique evolved from percutaneous techniques using a smaller tube, with the intention of providing access to the airway for prolonged periods, but without resorting to conventional tracheostomy. Although it is particularly effective for the management of postoperative sputum retention, particularly when placed electively, it is less reliable for airway access during long-term mechanical ventilation.

Cricothyroidotomy

Immediate access to the airway may be readily achieved by emergency cricothyroidotomy, particularly in the trauma setting when endotracheal intubation may not be possible. Initially, a needle (14-gauge cannula) may be inserted directly through the cricothyroid membrane into the airway, and connected to a high-pressure jet or bag ventilation. Otherwise, direct incision of the cricothyroid membrane may be performed and a tracheostomy tube inserted directly into the trachea. Cricothyroidotomy kits are available. An emergency cricothyroidotomy should be converted to a formal tracheostomy as soon as possible. Elective cricothyroidotomy for long-term airway management has remained controversial, although formal tracheostomy is now preferred. Complication rates up to 25% were reported for elective cricothyroidotomy, and in addition, several prospective studies have confirmed this procedure to be a risk factor for subglottic stenosis (4%) and voice change (15%).

Further reading

Golde AR, Irish JC, Gullane PJ. Tracheotomy. In: Pearson FG, Deslauriers J, Ginsberg RJ, Hiebert CA, McKneally MF, Urschel HC, eds. *Thoracic Surgery*. New York: Churchill Livingstone, 1995; 313.

Related topics of interest

TRAUMA

Simon Pickard, Alan G. Casson

The chest is frequently injured by both penetrating and blunt trauma, with a spectrum of injuries ranging from a simple rib fracture to exsanguinating vascular rupture. However, the majority of chest injuries do not require thoracotomy, and are managed by chest-tube drainage. Assessment of major intrathoracic organ damage should be performed concurrent with general resuscitation (airway, IV fluids, etc.) and the evaluation of other injuries (i.e. head, abdomen, muskuloskeletal).

Immediate life-threatening injuries

Evaluation and resuscitation of all traumatized patients is optimal when conducted in a systemic manner. Regardless of injury, a secure airway, breathing and circulation (ABC) must be achieved before attention to individual organ systems.

Airway

- A secure airway is the first priority of resuscitation.
- With appropiate stabilization of the cervical spine (always assumed to be unstable), this is generally achieved by endotracheal intubation.
- In a spontaneously breathing patient, nasotracheal intubation may be performed.
- A surgical airway (i.e. cricothyroidotomy, tracheostomy) is indicated in patients with significant maxillofacial (and cervical spine) injury.
- If there is suspected laryngotracheal injury, intubation over a flexible fiberoptic bronchoscope is ideal.

Initial evaluation

1. Physical examination
- Cyanosis: inadequate airway or failure of resuscitation.
- Respiratory effort: stridor suggests upper airway injury and may indicate unilateral chest movement, pneumothorax, hemothorax, bronchial rupture; paradoxical movement may indicate a flail chest; intercostal retractions suggests airway obstruction, respiratory distress.
- Pulse: irregularity suggests dysrhythmias; tachycardia may indicate hypovolemia, or cardiac tamponade; absent pulses may be indicative of major vessel injury or severe hypotension.
- Neck veins: distention suggests cardiac tamponade, tension pneumothorax or agitation.
- Subcutaneous emphysema: pneumothorax, pneumomediastinum, tracheobronchial injury.
- Lung and heart sounds.
- Examine the back of the chest as well as the front. Mark all penetrating (entry and exit) wounds.

2. *Radiology.* A portable CXR (A-P) is usually obtained initially. This should be examined in a systematic manner, with particular attention to the following.

- Position of all tubes and lines, including endotracheal tube, chest tubes, nasogastric tube and central venous lines.
- Pneumothorax: lung markings should reach the periphery. May be difficult to see if subcutaneous emphysema is present or film is overpenetrated.
- Mediastinal shift: suggesting a tension pneumo- or hemothorax.
- Opacification of a hemithorax: suggests hemothorax (or pulmonary fluid). May be subtle when supine, as fluid layers posteriorly.
- Mediastinal widening: suspicious for great vessel rupture. Look also for loss of contour of the aortic knob, depressed left mainstem bronchus, deviation of a nasogastric tube.
- Mediastinal emphysema. tracheobronchial or esophageal injury should be suspected.
- Rib fractures: upper rib fractures (especially first rib) make great vessel injury more probable.
- Ruptured diaphragm: may result in herniation of abdominal contents into the chest. A gas-filled loop of bowel may easily be mistaken for a pneumothorax.
- Heart contour: enlargement of the pericardium suggests pericardial hemorrhage.
- Pulmonary contusion: may not be apparent on the initial film; infiltration or opacification of the parenchyma developing over 24 hours is typical.
- Bullets or other foreign bodies should be documented.

Tension pneumothorax

Should be suspected in a patient with respiratory distress, hypotension, distended neck veins and hyperresonance of one hemithorax with absent breath sounds. The immediate placement of a needle to decompress the pleural space is life-saving, while definitive therapy is placement of a chest tube connected to underwater seal drainage.

Open pneumothorax

Usually results from a penetrating defect of the chest wall. Occlusion of the defect with placement of a chest tube is required prior to operative repair of the defect.

Flail chest

A flail segment results when multiple rib fractures separate a part of the chest wall, which moves paradoxically with breathing. The injury is recognized on physical examination. If respiratory distress is apparent, the patient should be intubated and ventilated initially, until the chest wall is stabilized. Young patients with small flail segments and no other major chest injuries may be managed with regional anesthesia (intercostal nerve blocks or epidural catheter) and vigorous physiotherapy.

Massive hemothorax

Massive bleeding into the thorax may initially tamponade the bleeding vessel. Placement of a chest tube may result in significant bleeding. If this is greater than 1500 ml, or is associated with hypotension, the chest tube should be clamped and a thoracotomy performed immediately (in the operating room) to control the source of bleeding. Ongoing bleeding through the chest tube (i.e. >300 ml/hour for 3 hours) is an indication for thoracotomy.

Pericardial tamponade

Hypotension, distended neck veins (or elevated CVP), an enlarged heart contour on the CXR, distant heart sounds, and pulsus paradoxus (a 10 mmHg drop in systolic blood pressure during inspiration, caused by decreased left ventricular stroke volume) should suggest pericardial tamponade. If echocardiography is not immediately available, pericardicentesis should be performed at once. A drainage catheter should be left in place. This is a temporary measure, and the patient should subsequently be taken to the operating room for definitive treatment (subxiphoid window or thoracotomy).

Emergency-room thoracotomy

Emergency-room thoracotomy is associated with high (>50%) mortality. It should be performed when shock persists despite adequate resuscitation. A left anterolateral approach is used, at the fourth interspace. The aim is to cross-clamp the descending thoracic aorta (to stop distal bleeding, and to increase coronary and cerebral perfusion), to evacuate the pericardium and to perform open cardiac massage.

Specific thoracic injuries

Further evaluation

After stabilization of the patient, and treatment of immediate life-threatening injuries, additional investigations may be required to identify specific thoracic injuries.

1. Radiology
- A P-A and lateral CXR (sitting or standing) may indicate the extent of pleural fluid (or blood), and permits evaluation of the superior mediastinum which may be widened (defined as >8 cm). Inspiratory/expiratory films may accentuate a small pneumothorax. Old films should be reviewed (if available).
- Oblique rib views: to demonstrate rib and sternal fractures.
- CT scanning. Provides a better evaluation of mediastinal structures, especially when intravenous and oral contrast is used.

- Esophageal contrast studies to diagnose esophageal disruption.
- Aortography: remains the definitive study to assess aortic rupture.

2. Arterial blood gases

3. EKG, echocardiography. Echocardiography is useful to diagnose accumulation of pericardial blood and to evaluate ventricular function. EKG monitoring is essential to detect dysrhythmias following myocardial contusion.

4. Bronchoscopy, thoracoscopy. Either investigation can be performed in the emergency room (if properly equipped), although it is often preferable to transfer the patient to the operating room. Bronchoscopy is performed to evaluate hemoptysis, and to diagnose suspected tracheobronchial injury. In an intubated patient, it is necessary to visualize the entire airway, and the endotracheal tube should be withdrawn temporarily so that the upper airway can be evaluated. Thoracoscopy may be used to evacuate pleural blood and to diagnose potential sites of bleeding (i.e. intercostal arteries, lung parenchyma) or diaphragmatic rupture.

Rib fracture

The significance of rib fractures relates to the degree of trauma transmitted to the chest wall and underlying viscera. Fractures of the upper ribs are associated with vascular injury, any rib fracture may be associated with pulmonary contusion. Lower rib fractures are associated with intra-abdominal (i.e. splenic, hepatic) injuries, sternal fractures with cardiac injury, and clavicular fractures with injuries of the subclavian vessels or brachial plexus. Control of pain, which may require epidural analgesia, is an essential component of management, especially in the elderly.

Pulmonary contusion, laceration

1. Contusion. Pulmonary contusion often follows blunt trauma, with associated rib fractures. It may not be apparent on initial CXR, but will be detected on serial radiographs (increasing infiltrates) and clinically (hypoxia, respiratory distress). Treatment is supportive. Progression to ARDS is associated with poor prognosis.

2. Laceration. Pulmonary lacerations may bleed briskly, often with an associated air leak. Initial management is chest-tube placement to evacuate of the pleural space, and permit expansion of the underlying lung. Ongoing bleeding, massive air leak and failure of the lung to expand are indications for thoracotomy and suture (or stapling) of the laceration. Concomittant bronchoscopy is indicated to evacuate blood from the airway and check for possible tracheal or bronchial injury.

Laryngotracheal injury	• Usually associated with other thoracic injuries and easily overlooked.

Laryngotracheal injury

- Usually associated with other thoracic injuries and easily overlooked.
- Immediate management is to secure an the airway (i.e. endotracheal intubation with a flexible bronchoscope or tracheostomy).
- Diagnosis is made by laryngoscopy/bronchoscopy.
- Indications for surgery include: (i) progressive subcutaneous emphysema, (ii) extensive mucosal lacerations with exposed cartilage, (iii) fracture of the laryngeal skeleton and (iv) penetrating wounds.

Tracheobronchial injury

This may occur with penetrating or blunt trauma, as a result of inhalation injury or as an iatrogenic injury caused by intubation. Most lacerations occur within 2–3 cm of the carina, with right mainstem bronchial injuries more frequent than left-sided injuries. The immediate presentation is usually mediastinal (and subcutaneous) emphysema, and pneumothorax with a massive air leak. The patient will deteriorate (i.e. become more dyspnoeic) if the underwater seal drainage system is connected to suction. Bronchoscopy is diagnostic, and immediate operative repair is required. The operative approach depends on the anatomic location of the injury and the presence of associated intrathoracic injuries requiring correction. The carina and a considerable amount of the left mainstem bronchus may be approached from a right thoracotomy. Small, chronic, or missed injuries may heal by granulation, and present with bronchial stenosis, leading to atelectasis, recurrent pneumonias and pulmonary sepsis. These may be repaired using bronchoplastic techniques, but occasionally pulmonary resection is required.

Diaphragmatic injury

1. Acute blunt rupture. This follows abdominal or thoracic trauma, which results in a pressure gradient between each cavity. It is most commonly the result of rapid deceleration. Both sides are affected equally, but left-sided injuries are diagnosed more frequently. The rupture results in herniation of the abdominal viscera into the chest, which may initially cause in cardiorespiratory compromise. Initial management is with nasogastric intubation, avoidance of chest-tube placement and surgical repair. Laparotomy is preferred in view of the associated abdominal injuries (seen in over 90% of patients).

2. Acute penetrating injury. These are generally smaller defects than seen with blunt rupture and immediate herniation is rare. Associated abdominal injuries are also common, and often dominate the initial clinical presentation. At laparotomy, both hemi-diaphragms should be examined carefully, and repaired.

3. Chronic diaphragmatic hernia. Approximately 10–20% of acute diaphragmatic injuries (especially the smaller, penetrating injuries) are missed. The negative pleuroperitoneal gradient is an important factor in the development of chronic herniation, which may result in incarceration, strangulation, GI obstruction or respiratory compromise. Asymptomatic herniae may be discovered on incidental CXR. Elective repair is indicated, using a transthoracic approach to lyse adhesions safely.

Cardiac trauma

Penetrating or blunt chest trauma may involve the heart. The right ventricle, situated substernally, is most vulnerable to injury. Lacerations of cardiac chambers require direct operative repair. Associated septal defects and valvular injuries are frequent with blunt trauma, but rarely require immediate surgical correction. Cardiac contusion should be managed like a myocardial infarction, as a comparable spectrum of complications may develop. Injuries of the great vessels (i.e. aorta, pulmonary artery and vein) are repaired by direct suture. Occasionally, cardiopulmonary bypass may be required.

Esophageal injury

- Uncommon injuries; the cervical esophagus is most frequently involved.
- Diagnosis is made with contrast esophagography and endoscopy.
- Exploration of all injuries is recommended. Primary repair (with adequate local drainage) is preferred, but esophageal diversion (i.e. cervical spit fistula, mediastinal drainage, gastrostomy, feeding jejunostomy) or resection may be required. Reconstruction is performed as a second, staged, procedure.

Chylothorax

- A result of thoracic duct injury at any level.
- Presents as a persistent pleural collection, or as chyle drainage through an indwelling chest tube.
- See 'Chylothorax', p. 52.

Traumatic asphyxia

- Results from prolonged chest compression, against a closed glottis. This leads to increased intrathoracic venous pressure, which is transmitted to the head and neck.
- Characterized by facial cyanosis (also may involve the upper torso), edema, and disorientation which improves within 24 hours.
- Management is that of associated thoracic injuries.

Further reading

Baxter BT, Moore EE, Cleveland HC. Emergency department thoracotomy following injury: critical determinants for survival. *World Journal of Surgery*, 1988; **12**: 671.

Cogbill TH, Landercasper J. Injury to the chest wall. In: Moore EE, Mattox KL, Feliciano DV, eds. *Trauma,* 2nd edn. Norwalk: Appleton and Lange, 1991; 327.

Eddy CA, Carrico CJ, Rusch VW. Injury to the lung and pleura. In: Moore EE, Mattox KL, Feliciano DV, eds. *Trauma,* 2nd edn. Norwalk: Appleton and Lange, 1991; 358.

Lang-Lazdunski L, Mouroux J, Pons F, Grosdidier G, Martinod E, Elkaim D, Azorin J, Jancovici R. Role of videothoracoscopy in chest trauma. *Annals of Thoracic Surgery,* 1997; **63:** 324.

Pate JW. Tracheobronchial and esophageal injuries. *Surgery Clinics in North America,* 1989; **69:** 1.

Schaefer SD. The acute management of laryngeal trauma: a 27 year experience. *Archives of Otolaryngology and Head and Neck Surgery,* 1992; **118:** 598.

Stewart KC, Urschel JD, Naki SS, Gelfand ET, Hamilton SM. Pulmonary resection for lung trauma. *Annals of Thoracic Surgery,* 1997; **63:** 1587.

Symbias PN, Justicz AG, Ricketts RR. Rupture of the airways from blunt trauma: treatment of complex injuries. *Annals of Thoracic Surgery,* 1992; **54:** 177.

Related topics of interest

TUBERCULOSIS

Simon Pickard, Alan G. Casson

Although the field of general thoracic surgery had its foundations based on surgery for pulmonary tuberculosis, the need for surgical management of this disease diminished with the advent of effective chemotherapy. However, tuberculosis remains a problem worldwide, and in recent years the incidence of pulmonary tuberculosis has increased in developed countries, especially in immunocompromised patients. Unfortunately, many new cases appear to be resistant to first-line drugs, and the emergence of multidrug-resistant *Mycobacterium tuberculosis*, and mycobacteria other than tuberculosis (atypical), has led to additional patients requiring surgical management.

Microbiology

1. Mycobacterium tuberculosis
- A non-sporing bacillus; an obligate anaerobe.
- Extremely virulent; capable of invading normal tissues.
- High lipid content in the cell wall results in acid-fast staining (Ziehl–Neilsen). Smears may be used to estimate infectious load or response to therapy.
- Culture of specimens is essential for accurate bacteriologic diagnosis. These organisms are characteristically slow growing, and culture (and drug sensitivity) may take up to 6 weeks. Newer techniques (PCR-based) may allow more rapid detection.

2. Atypical tuberculosis. Mycobacteria other than tuberculosis are generally named after their source or site of origin: *M. avium-intracellulare, M. leprai, M. bovis, M. xenopi, M. kansaii,* etc. These organisms are found free in the environment, have characteristic growth patterns in culture, are generally less virulent than *M. tuberculosis*, and tend to invade hosts with abnormalities of the underlying lung.

Pathology

1. Stage I. Primary (childhood) tuberculosis follows airborne infection of the bronchial tree, resulting in a variable host response. Overwhelming infection may occur in immunocompromised individuals. In the absence of tuberculin sensitivity, the disease does not progress (tuberculin test remains negative). Eventual sensitivity to the tubercule results in a positive tuberculin test, and the disease resolves as an insignificant scar (Ghon complex).

2. Stage II. Characterized by lymphatic or hematogenous infection, resulting in miliary tuberculosis.

3. Stage III. Acquisition of a marked sensitivity to the tubercule bacillus results in pulmonary reinfection (exogenous or endogenous), and destructive, cavitary disease in adults.

Clinical presentation	As the majority of patients present with nonspecific symptoms (i.e. malaise, anorexia, fever, cough, weight loss, etc.), a high index of suspicion must be maintained. This is especially true for patients with previous exposure, with underlying lung disease (i.e. bronchiectasis), with associated medical diseases (i.e. diabetes or immunosuppression) and who are homeless.
Diagnosis	• Bacteriologic culture and sensitivity. Specimens may be obtained from sputum, bronchial washings, pleural biopsy, lymph node aspirate or biopsy. • Tuberculin skin testing (i.e. Mantoux or Heaf tests). Conversion from negative to positive indicates recent infection. False negative tests may be seen in immunosuppressed individuals. • Chest X-ray, or CT, to define the extent of pulmonary parenchymal lesions.
Management	*1. General.* An index of population health, nutrition, etc. As this disease is highly contagious, attention should be given to established infectious control measures. *2. Medical.* First-line therapy is medical. Multidrug therapy may be started empirically, and then modified once culture and sensitivity information are available. The duration and type of therapy is revised frequently, and current recommendations should be followed. *3. Surgical.* Surgery may be considered for the following: • For diagnosis [i.e. wedge excision of a solitary peripheral nodule (tuberculoma)]. • Massive hemoptysis (tuberculosis is the most common cause of massive hemoptysis). • Bronchopleural fistula with tuberulous empyema. • Trapped lung following empyema (i.e. decortication). • Persistent localized infection in destroyed lung or distal to bronchostenosis. • An open, culture-negative, cavity (>2 cm) in a young patient. • Localized disease resulting from atypical multidrug-resistant organisms.
Technical considerations	*1. Preoperative.* Assessment (and correction) of the following is essential: • Pulmonary function (i.e. pulmonary function studies, ventilation–perfusion scanning). • Nutrition. • Extent of disease (CT scanning, bronchoscopy). • Preoperative chemotherapy (for at least 2 weeks).

2. *Intraoperative*
- Double-lumen endotracheal intubation or a bronchial blocker is used to prevent contamination of the non-operated lung through the bronchial tree. With modern intubation techniques, thoracotomy in a prone position (rather than the standard lateral position) is no longer utilized.
- Extrapleural dissection is often required.
- Muscle flaps are used frequently to reinforce bronchial suture lines and to obliterate pleural spaces.
- All diseased lung tissue is removed.
- Pleuropneumonectomy may be required for empyema with bronchopleural fistula.

3. *Postoperative.* The most serious postoperative complication is a bronchopleural fistula. This is more common on the right side, and is generally related to ongoing bacteriologic contamination. Further flap rotation, or occasionally collapse therapy (thoracoplasty), may be necessary for ultimate resolution.

Further reading

Pomerantz M. Surgery for tuberculosis. *Chest Surgery Clinics of North America,* 1993; **3:** 723.
Treasure RL, Seaworth BJ. Current role of surgery in mycobacterium tuberculosis. *Annals of Thoracic Surgery,* 1995; **59:** 1405.

Related topics of interest

Bronchopleural fistula (p. 29)
Empyema (p. 75)
Hemoptysis (massive) (p. 129)

VIDEO-ASSISTED THORACOSCOPIC SURGERY

Gail Darling

Minimally invasive surgical approaches to the chest (i.e. thoracoscopy, mediastinoscopy, mediastinotomy) have been widely used in thoracic surgical practice for years. Technologic developments, and widespread availability of video imaging in the late 1980s, expanded thoracoscopy into video-assisted thoracoscopic surgery (VATS), enhancing both diagnostic and therapeutic applications. The potential advantages of this approach are related to the minimally invasive nature of this procedure, potentially resulting in less postoperative pain, respiratory dysfunction and hospitalization. It should be remembered that VATS represents only an approach to the thoracic cavity, and that adherence to the same surgical principles as for open procedures, is mandatory. Conversion of a VATS procedure to an open procedure should not be viewed as a technical failure, but rather an exercise of judgement. This section reviews VATS in general, then summarizes specific procedures.

Indications for VATS   In current clinical practice, VATS is believed to be the preferred (or an accepted) approach for the following procedures.

1. Generally accepted diagnostic indications
- Diagnosis of pleural effusions.
- Pleural biopsy.
- Wedge resection of lung for diagnosis of diffuse lung infiltrates or peripheral nodules.
- Biopsy of mediastinal masses.

2. Generally accepted therapeutic indications
- Pleurodesis (mechanical, chemical) or pleurectomy for malignant pleural effusions.
- Resection of apical pleural blebs for spontaneous pneumothorax.
- Evacuation of early empyema.
- Pericardial window.
- Excision of esophageal leiomyomas.
- Esophageal myotomy.
- Thoracic sympathectomy.

3. Evolving indications
- Excision of posterior mediastinal masses.
- Lung volume reduction surgery.
- Wedge resection of small peripheral lung tumors in selected patients with limited lung function.
- Decortication of empyemas.
- Staging esophageal cancer.
- Spinal surgery (disk disease, spinal abcess).
- Exploration for trauma.

4. Controversial or highly experimental indications
- Formal pulmonary resections (i.e. lobectomy, pneumonectomy) for cancer.
- Resection of eosphageal cancer.

5. Contraindications
- Obliterated pleural space (i.e. history of tuberculosis, empyema).
- Inability to tolerate single-lung anesthesia.
- Respiratory failure requiring mechanical ventilation particularly if high airway pressures or PEEP.
- Contralateral pneumonectomy.

Operative technique

1. Preoperative assessment. As for any general thoracic procedure: see 'Preoperative assessment for thoracic surgery', p. 212.

2. Anesthesia
- General anesthesia.
- Single-lung anesthesia is required (i.e. double-lumen endotracheal tube or bronchial blocker).
- Usual intraoperative monitoring, etc.: see 'Anesthesia for thoracic surgery', p. 8.

3. Equipment
- Open thoracotomy set-up should be readily available.
- Rigid thoracoscope (0 or 30°), or hybrid with operating channel.
- Light source: high intensity (xenon or metal halide) video monitor, camera, VCR.
- Thoracoports (10 or 12 mm): may be optional.
- Electrocautery (monopolar).
- Smoke evacuator (especially if laser used).
- Instruments: dedicated VATS instruments, laparoscopic instruments, standard (nonendoscopic) instruments, endoscopic staplers, clip appliers, endoscissors and specimen bags.

4. Set-up. The monitor(s) should be opposite the surgeon/ assistant, orientated in the direction of surgery, to avoid a mirror-imaging effect. The port position is critical. The camera port is usually guided by the specific procedure and expected pathology. Subsequent ports are placed under direct vision, in the line of a standard thoracotomy incision (where possible), with triangulation of the port sites to minimize obstruction within the operative field. Ports are placed at a distance from the target area to facilitate instrumentation within the thoracic cavity.

5. *Postoperative management.* As for any thoracic surgical procedure: see 'Postoperative management and complications', p. 206.

Pulmonary resections

VATS is primarily used for diagnostic lung biopsy. It is currently not an acceptable technique for formal lung resection of cancer. However, in selected patients with limited pulmonary reserve, a wedge excision of a T1N0 non-small cell lung carcinoma may be performed as a compromise procedure. VATS is not recommended for the excision of metastatic nodules, which may be difficult to localize (not palpable with VATS), and are often more numerous than predicted by preoperative CT scanning.

Resection of apical blebs

VATS is used widely to resect apical blebs resulting in primary recurrent pneumothorax, especially combined with pleural abrasion or parietal pleurectomy. Its advantage over axillary thoracotomy is questionable. Pneumonthorax secondary to bullous disease is more difficult to treat in view of the diffuse nature of the disease, and identification of the disrupted bullae with the lung collapsed.

Pleural procedures

- Diagnosis of pleural masses: for suspected mesothelioma, use only one port to limit sites where tumor may grow through chest wall.
- Diagnosis and management of pleural effusions: drain the effusion completely, break up fluid loculations, extensive pleural biopsies, assess lung expansion and, if complete, proceed with pleurodesis.
- Management of early empyema: evacuate all pleural fluid (i.e. infected effusion, pus, clotted hemothorax), assess lung re-expansion, and debride fibrin and loculations.

Mediastinal surgery

- Staging of lung cancer, particularly assessment of nodes not accessible by cervical mediastinoscopy (subaortic, inferior pulmonary ligament, posterior subcarinal).
- Useful for biopsy/resection of various cysts and benign lesions.

Thoracic sympathectomy

- Excellent visualization of the sympathetic chain makes VATS an ideal approach.
- Results are best for hyperhidrosis; variable for reflex sympathetic dystrophy.
- Avoid use of cautery near stellate ganglion to avoid Horner's syndrome.

Esophageal surgery

- Role in staging and excision of esophageal carcinoma is under evaluation.
- A suitable approach for excision of benign tumors (i.e. leiomyoma).

- When VATS myotomy is performed for achalasia (or other motor disorders), simultaneous esophagogastroscopy is useful to localize the esophagogastric junction, and to exclude mucosal damage at the termination of the procedure.

Laparoscopic anti-reflux surgery. General thoracic surgeons with an esophageal interest should be familiar with laparoscopic anti-reflux surgery. The preoperative investigations and indications for surgery are the same as for open approaches. The success of any transabdominal (including laparoscopic) approach requires an adequate length of intra-abdominal esophagus around which a fundoplication is performed. After abdominal insufflation, the camera port is placed halfway between umbilicus and xiphoid, a 30° scope provides excellent visualization. The hiatus is closed using interrupted non-absorbable sutures, with a bougie (>50 F) in the esophagus. Several short gastrics are usually ligated (or divided using the harmonic scalpel) to mobilize the fundus for a tension-free wrap. A 2–3 cm fundoplication (Nissen, 360°) is performed with a large bougie in place.

Further reading

Brown WT, ed. *Atlas of Video-Assisted Thoracic Surgery*. Philadelphia: WB Saunders, 1994.

Landreneau RJ, Mack MJ, Dowling RD, Luketich JD, Keenan RJ, Ferson PF, Hazelrigg SR. The role of thoracoscopy in lung cancer management. *Chest,* 1998; **113 (Suppl.):** 6S.

Lewis RJ, ed. Video-assisted thoracic surgery. *Chest Surgery Clinics of North America,* 1993, **3:** 2.

Lewis RJ, Caccavale RJ, Sisler GE. Video-assisted thoracic surgery. In: Pearson FG, Deslauriers J, Ginsberg RJ, Hiebert CA, McKneally MF, Urschel HC, eds. *Thoracic Surgery.* New York: Churchill Livingstone, 1995; 917.

Mack MJ, Scruggs GR, Kelly KM, Shennib H, Landreneau RJ. Video-assisted thoracic surgery: has technology found its place? *Annals of Thoracic Surgery,* 1997; **64:** 211.

Peters JH. Laparoscopy and thoracoscopy of the esophagus: what's new? *Diseases of the Esophagus,* 1997; **10:** 279.

Yim APC, Liu HP, Hazelrigg SR, Izzat MB, Fung ALK, Boley TM, Magee MJ. Thoroscopic operations on reoperated chests. *Annals of Thoracic Surgery,* 1998; **65:** 328.

Related topics of interest

INDEX